Some Crawl and Never Walk

by
Celestine Tate

D0791788

DORRANCE PUBLISHING CO., INC.
PITTSBURGH, PENNSYLVANIA 15222

ISBN # 0-8059-3652-1
Printed in the United States of America

Second Printing

For information or to order additional books, please write:
Dorrance Publishing Co., Inc.
643 Smithfield Street
Pittsburgh, Pennsylvania 15222
U.S.A.

Even as a young child, I dreamed about someday being able to shout loud enough for everyone to hear, "Hey, even the most severely handicapped can contribute to your life!" I feel that I have coped successfully with unique problems which others who have difficulties not half as severe might solve through knowledge and experience. The solutions to my problems were the result of self–control, determination, and self–respect.

I am very happy that I have found the way to write this book. It would not have been possible without the help of my friend, Sally Sharp; my grandparents, Mr. and Mrs. Omega Leach; and Cherrie, who is not only a great woman, but who has been a positive influence on my life. So, because of them and all mankind, I hope that this book will help answer in some small way to those who ask, "Why me?"

I would also like to thank Mr. Holyfield for pushing me in the right direction, and Mr. Ron Bell for being his agent. Because of the two of them, I know this will be a better world in which to live.

"Never cry about not being able to walk because I have a plan for you. You will grow up and have children, and be known all over the world. You will come into contact with good people and bad people. Be strong for I will always be with you."

—Coming from the Lord

Contents

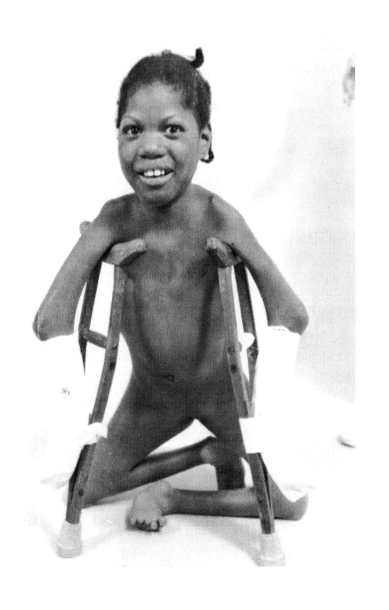

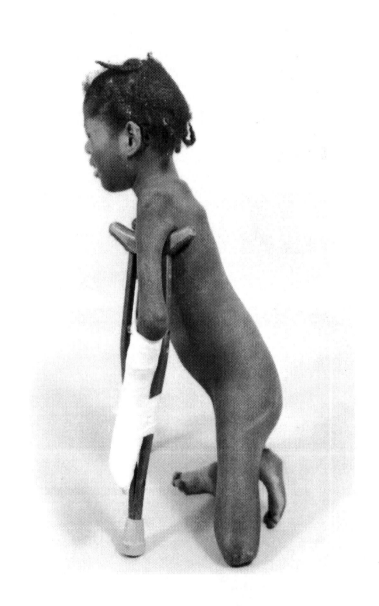

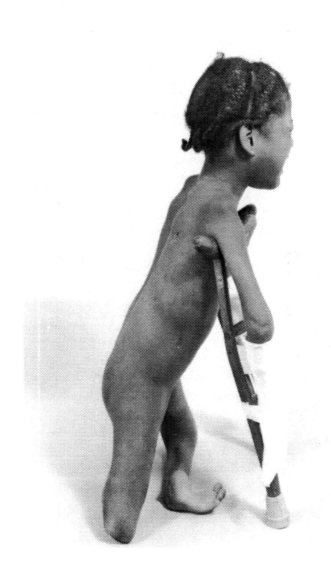

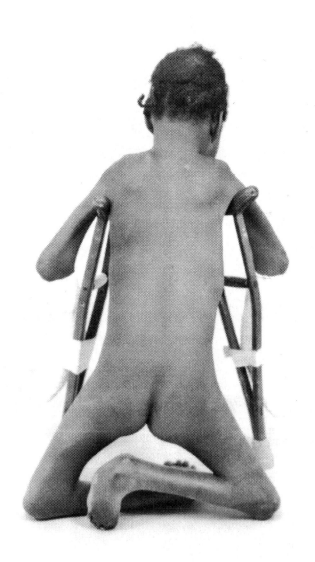

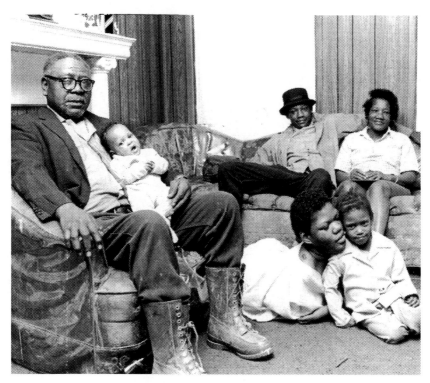

Reprinted by permission of JET Magazine,
© 1976, Johnson Publishing Company, Inc.

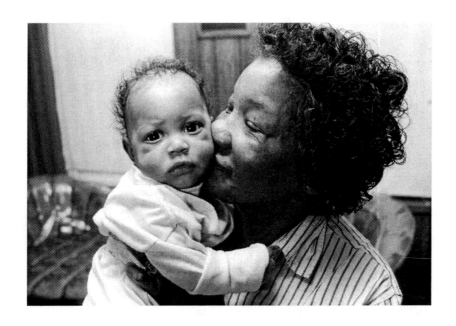

Reprinted by permission of JET Magazine,
© 1976, Johnson Publishing Company, Inc.

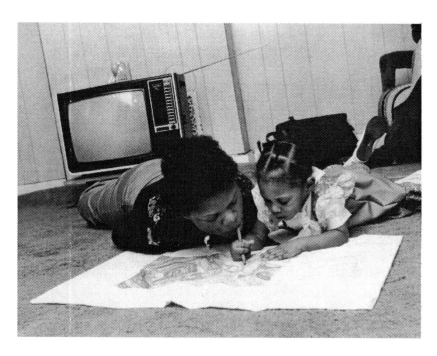

Reprinted by permission of JET Magazine,
© 1976, Johnson Publishing Company, Inc.

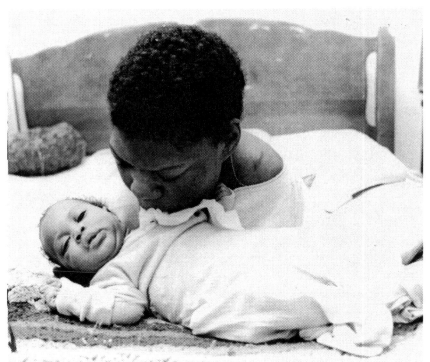

Reprinted by permission of JET Magazine,
© 1976, Johnson Publishing Company, Inc.

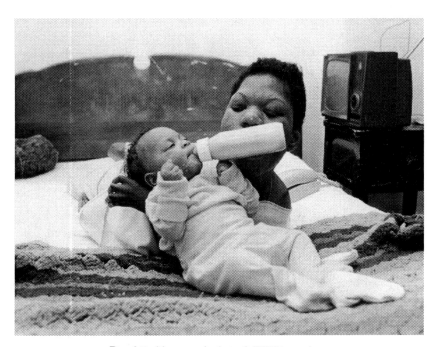
Reprinted by permission of JET Magazine,
© 1976, Johnson Publishing Company, Inc.

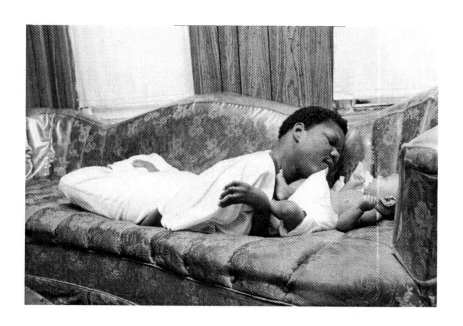

ALL BY OURSELVES

I was born in a Philadelphia hospital at 10:45 P.M. on Thursday, October 15, 1955. My mother, Frances Tate, was told beforehand that I would have medical problems because she had tried to abort me during the early months of her pregnancy.

I was born with my left arm and both legs folded backward, in a reverse lotus position. My right hand was in my mouth. In order to remove it, the arm was broken surgically, then reset. And so all my limbs would be forever useless. I weighed one pound, six ounces and was declared, "the smallest infant that ever survived at that time." To this day, my nickname is Teeny.

I was fed through my nose in an incubator for the first three months of my life. Years later I was told that the hospital staff had discussed with my mother the possibility of her selling me to the hospital for experimental purposes. She declined the offer because, a former friend explained, "She felt that you must have been her punishment for trying to abort you." She was only sixteen years old, and I was the first of her three children.

For the next six years, I remained with my mother in North Philadelphia on 17th and Montgomery Avenue. It was an old three-story house.

By the age of three, my awareness of being handicapped increased steadily. This was probably due to my sister, Maggie, who was born a mere eleven months after me. She weighed five pounds, ten ounces at birth, and she was completely normal. Still, we were very close.

I remember Maggie playing, running, skipping, and jumping. I remember wondering *"Why can't I do the same?"* So one day I asked, "Mom, why can't I play like Maggie?"

She answered calmly, "God put you like that because he wanted to see how people would treat you all your life."

I was puzzled. "Does this mean I'll be like this all the time?" She hesitated, then said, "No, when you get to be a lady, you'll walk."

I remembered that previous summer, when I was four, my father's mother, who we called "Momma," had taught me about God and so I understood my mother's words.

I recalled my father's mother sitting on her bed next to me one Sunday afternoon reading a little black book. She asked, "Teeny, does Frances read the Bible to you and Maggie?"

I replied, "I don't know! Is it like, *"Fun With Dick and Jane?"* She was apparently upset.

"This little black book tells us all we need to know about God. We Baptists keep our faith in God."

I asked, "So why don't we invite God to dinner?"

She laughed, "God can't come to dinner. He's in heaven."

"Where's that, Momma?"

"Some people say that heaven is up there in the sky."

"If I could stand outside, Momma, would I be able to see Him?"

"No, child. God is a spirit. He's something wonderful, but you can't see Him. You have to have faith that He is here with you right now, and always."

"Tell me, Momma, what does God do?"

"God is your creator. He made you and Maggie and everyone and everything in the world. As long as you believe in Him and say your prayers, He will take care of you."

Momma opened that little black book. "I am going to read the 23rd Psalm." She proceeded quietly, "The Lord is my shepherd, I shall not want...."

"I listened and felt hope.

My Momma. She was only fifty–two at the time and a mere five–feet–four. She had long, straight, grey hair. She was a great cook who gave Maggie and me the finest meals of our childhood. After all she'd had seven children of her own to cook for. We lived for our visits to see this kind woman.

As usual our mother went out and left Maggie and me all alone. She locked us in her bedroom with one gallon of water, four boiled eggs, a loaf of bread, and four hotdogs. She said, "I'll be back in an hour."

I was five years old and Maggie was four. We looked at the television. Maggie ate the eggs and hotdogs and most of the bread. Finally she cried, "Oh, I'm scared. It's getting dark. Where's Mom?"

Remembering that I was Big Sis, I told her, "Don't cry, Mom will be right back." Maggie laid on my back and fell asleep.

Since Maggie ate a lot, I had finally given her even the last of the bread. I did not eat that day. I remained awake. Then I began to hear noises. *Mom's coming home*, I thought. But the bedroom door did not unlock. Only the rats crawled around on the floor. Would they eat me? I was so hungry that I decided, "Humph! I might eat them!" Finally, I fell asleep.

Maggie woke me up with, "I'm hungry! Mommy hasn't come home yet, and it's daytime again. Where is she, Teeny?"

I thought quickly, then said, "Mommy's sick. She had to go to the doctor. She'll be back in awhile."

So Maggie continued to urinate in the bucket Mom had left. She helped me as I leaned over and used the bucket, too.

Television kept us company that whole long day. Mom didn't come back. At about six P.M., Maggie went to the window and watched the snow on the ground on that cold second night alone. She started to cry. "It's getting dark again!"

And the television blew out. By eight P.M., Maggie had cried herself to sleep, laying on my back.

I lay there and wondered, "Where's Mom? It's two days now, and Maggie's hungry."

Suddenly my handicap didn't seem so important. I thought, *What will I do if Mom doesn't come home tomorrow? If I could walk, I would go get help. Maggie's too young to go out in the snow all by herself. Besides her coat is not in here and she might catch a cold.*

I cried, very quietly, so that Maggie wouldn't notice. I was afraid she would starve to death. Then I slept.

On the third morning, Maggie woke up playing. Her whole attitude had changed. The burden of her being hungry was lifted from me for awhile. She opened a dresser drawer and finally lifted something up. "A screwdriver." Then something came to me. I said, "Stick it in the lock, then pull the door fast." She did so. The door opened! We were free!

"Maggie, go see what's in the kitchen to eat!" Since we were on the second floor, she had to go downstairs.

She returned and said, "There's a box of cereal and no milk, bologna, and no bread." She munched on the bologna as she spoke. I wanted some.

But she asked worriedly, "Teeny, why is the couch, the record player, and the TV, and the rug, and the fish tank all gone?"

I thought, *Some of the neighborhood dope addicts took 'em. So...that was the noise I heard the other night when I thought Mom had come home.*

Maggie went down to get the box of cereal for me. Then I heard voices. Who was Maggie talking to? She came up the stairs crying.

"What's wrong, Maggie?"

"Mommy hit me for spilling the cereal...."

Whew! At least she was home again. I wondered, *How can Mom hit Maggie for being hungry after she's been gone so long?*

She came up the stairs with her girlfriend, Sandy. I asked, "Mom, where have you been?"

3

She answered as though I had no business asking, "Out of town, Teeny."

Sandy asked, "How do you and Maggie feel?"

My sister and I answered together, "Hungry."

Mom had a bag filled with Chinese food and we knew that we were going to get some.

Sandy went into the bathroom and ran bath water. I thought, *Finally we're going to get a bath. I feel dirty. Wish I could wash Maggie and me without needing anybody.*

Sandy washed Maggie as Mom undressed in the adjoining bedroom. Suddenly Mom yelled angrily, "Why was the damn door open? Where's all my furniture? Teeny, if you don't tell me right now I'm going to beat y'r ass!"

She sat on the side of my bed, rolled her funny–looking cigarette, and demanded, "Answer me! Did Maggie let somebody in here?"

"...Er, er, two nights ago I heard a noise...but...but nobody came up. I thought it was you. We didn't know that the furniture was gone 'til just now."

"It must have been those dope addicts," I said.

"What d' you know about dope addicts?"

"I heard you and Sandy talk about them."

She was silent as Maggie and Sandy played in the bathroom. Then Maggie ran into the bedroom, wet and naked. She was so glad Mom was home. I was glad for her sake, and my sake for I was so hungry.

Mom picked me up and took me into the bathroom. She laid me on the table there, removed my clothes and placed me in the tub. Then she squirted soap all over me, "Give yourself a bath!"

I moved around, splashing back and forth, up and down in the water, determined to do it myself. Then Mom came back and rinsed me off. She returned me to the bedroom, where Maggie was already eating and grinning and looking so happy.

Right then, although I was only five, I knew that I had to live, not for myself, but for my sister.

At that moment, I started to cry. I was so hungry, and Mom would usually feed me any other time. I couldn't figure out why she was being so hard on me now.

Suddenly a bright light beamed through the window covering the whole room. It was so bright, I had to hold my head down. I remembered telling Maggie to close her eyes tight.

Then I heard a voice. I lifted my head and opened my eyes.

My sister had a spoonful of Chinese food coming towards her mouth and she appeared to be awake, but yet when I called her, she didn't answer me.

My mother was sitting at her vanity table combing her long, curly hair, and she was also frozen.

Sandy, who was sitting in front of the TV, was as stiff as a board.

Then suddenly an image appeared on the wall. It was an image of a man in the form of a light.

He didn't exactly have a voice, but he sent the beam of light to my head. This beam of light told me what my life would be like.

He said, "Never cry about being handicapped because I have a plan for you. You will grow up and have children, then be married, and be known all over the world. You will come into contact with both good and bad people. Be strong, for I will always be with you."

He told me I was filled with love, and to never cry about the condition I was in, and to write a book that would support myself and Maggie.

The light got bright again. I held my head down, it was too bright for my eyes.

Suddenly I heard Maggie, Sandy, and Mom and all was back to normal. I wanted to tell them what had happened to me, but something inside kept me from it.

I laid and cried, wondering, *How am I going to eat? I am so hungry.*

Mom put on my nightgown, and Sandy fixed my food. Sandy sat it in front of me on the bed. I waited for her to feed me, but Mom said, "Let her feed herself."

That wonderful Chinese food was getting cold. Desperately I pulled the plate close to my mouth with my tongue. I repeated the action faster and faster. The food surely tasted good. *Gee, it's fun to be able to do it all by myself!* I thought.

Maggie watched me. Then she started to eat with her mouth, too. I thought it was cute, but Mom slapped Maggie in the face and yelled, "Your sister can't help the way she eats. You eat the way you've been taught to eat!"

Maggie picked up her fork. Mom sighed. She walked up to Sandy and put her arms around her neck. She kissed her like I'd seen women kiss men on TV as Sandy rubbed her fingers through my mother's long, curly hair. Sandy asked, "Frances, when can I move in?"

Mom answered softly, "You're not leaving," and they started to kiss just like before.

After we ate, Mom kicked the television. It worked again! Maggie wanted to watch "The Beverly Hillbillies," but I wanted to see "Peyton Place."

"Neither one of you gonna see any TV. You're goin' to bed," Mom said. She picked me up, carried me into our bedroom and laid me on my twin bed. Maggie followed. There were two beds, but Maggie, as usual, crept in with me anyway. And, as usual, she asked me to help her say her prayers as Momma had taught us.

"Now I lay me down to sleep, I pray the Lord my soul to keep. If I should die before I wake, I pray the Lord my soul to take. God bless Mommy, Daddy, and everybody in the whole world. Amen."

Of course Maggie had to add, "And God Bless Lady."
(Lady was our little dog, so named because of my hopes of
"walking when I was a lady.")

Maggie wouldn't go to sleep. She was on another questioning spree.
"Teeny, where's Daddy? How come he hasn't come to see us in so long?"

I replied, as I had often before, "Daddy's busy on his new job. He'll
be here to see us as soon as he can. You know he loves us."

Maggie continued, "Wish we could live with Daddy instead of here
with Mommy. Why can't we, Teeny?"

"Like I said, Maggie, Daddy's very busy, and Mom loves us and
would miss us if we left her."

"Why doesn't Daddy live here with us anymore?" my little sister
persisted.

"Because Mom has friends Daddy doesn't like, so he can't stay."

"But why is Sandy sleeping on Daddy's side of the bed now?"

As I racked my brain for another excuse, I looked over. Maggie had
fallen asleep. I was left with the job of answering her questions to myself.

And then there was a loud whimpering from the adjoining bedroom.
I turned over and looked through the crack in the door. The steady
whimpering came from Mom. Mom kept repeating, "Sandy, I love you.
Sandy, I love you." Sandy's face was between my mother's legs.

Very carefully I took the cover up and pulled it over my little sister's
head with my mouth. I wished I was able to stick my fingers in my ears
so I did not hear those sounds. I knew those sounds would never leave
my mind.

The only way I was finally able to get to sleep was to promise myself
to tell Daddy about Mom and Sandy the next time he visited.

The next morning, Mom's voice awakened me. "It's time to get
dressed, Teeny. I'm going to buy you and Maggie some new clothes
today."

Maggie opened her eyes and yelped, "Whee, a coat! Now I can go out!"

Mom said, "You can wear your coat from last year 'til you get a new
one."

Sandy came in with a bright, "Good morning!" I turned toward the
wall. All I knew was that I didn't want to see her face. So Sandy dressed
Maggie, and Mom dressed me.

Mom said, "Sandy, there's not a drop of food in the house."

Sandy promised, "I'll go shopping after we get the kids' things." She
went into the other bedroom and took off her man's shorts. Then she put
on some dungarees and an old work shirt similar to the one my
grandfather wore on his construction job.

Mom said, "Sandy will take us all out for breakfast." Maggie was
happy, but I didn't want to go anywhere with that woman. When she
took Maggie with her to get the car, I asked, "Mom, is Sandy always
gonna live with us? Is she, is she?"

"Why, don't you like Sandy?"

"No," I pouted.

"Why, what did Sandy ever do to you?"

"She didn't do anything to me, but I saw what she did to you last night."

"You don't understand, Teeny. I love Sandy." Before I could say anything else, Sandy and Maggie returned.

"Forget it now," Mom said. She picked me up, carried me downstairs, and put my coat on.

Sandy picked me up. I bit her. I kept biting her. Mom grabbed me and said, "That girl's just being hateful." (She had to say something.) "I'll carry her."

Sandy shook her head, "I don't know why she doesn't like me. I never did anything wrong to her." She held Mom's arm as we went out the door and down the outside stairs. She opened the car door and helped Mom put me in the back seat. She kept complaining, "I don't know what's wrong. I never did nothing to her."

Mom wanted to drive, but Sandy said, "You're not wrecking my new car."

"My mother argued, "I've been driving for two years now."

Sandy settled the question, "I've been driving since 1950, and it's 1961 now. So I'll drive." She got behind the wheel and, we went to Tony's, a nearby Bar and Grill which sold food.

Sandy and Mom helped me into that place, and I sat on Mom's lap. She asked, "What do you want to eat, Teeny?" I turned and asked Maggie the same question. Maggie said, "Eggs and milk." So Sandy took Maggie to the counter, and Mom asked me, "Do you want some pancakes?"

"Yes, and bacon, too."

So Sandy bought Maggie and me our food. Two things were strange; neither Mom nor Sandy ate, Mom fed me in the restaurant, she wouldn't feed me at home. I didn't understand.

As we started to leave the restaurant, I noticed everyone staring at me. Were they looking because my mother was so pretty, or were they looking at me in her arms?

Maggie pouted and asked a man standing next to us, "What you looking at?"

Sandy tugged her hand and said, "Shut up!"

Then I knew. They were looking at me.

I wanted to cry, but remembered what Mom had said about God making me this way to see how people would treat me. After all our grandmother, Momma, had taught me how wonderful God was. And so I didn't cry. I looked forward to the fulfillment of my mother's promise; "walking when I was a lady."

We got back into the car and Sandy asked, "Where do you want to go shopping, Cradwick's or Jeckler's Kiddie Shop?"

Mom said, "Jeckler's Kiddie Shop. There's not too many people there, so Teeny won't be stared at too much."

We stopped at a street light, and Mom hollered out the window, "Bill, come here!" Sandy looked at her angrily. A tall, thirty–five–year old, well–dressed black man came to the car.

She asked excitedly, "Got anything hot to sell?"

The stranger replied, "Not right now, but I'll let you know, Frances."

I almost fell off Mom's lap as Sandy revved up the motor and cut around the corner. "How long you been knowing that damn pimp?" she asked.

"Oh, he's just an old neighborhood friend," Mom answered.

Sandy said worriedly, "We're gonna have to make some money because your habit's so expensive."

After a short drive, she turned up a long driveway to the rear of an old house. She asked, "How much do you want?"

Mom said, "Forty–five cents."

"Are you gonna sell it or smoke it yourself?"

"Both," Mom said.

"So why do you need a whole ounce?"

"If you're gonna be so cheap, I'll get another man!" Mom told her.

Sandy got out of the car and went into the house without another word.

Mom called to Maggie who was seated in the back. Maggie didn't answer.

"She's probably sleeping," I said.

Mom smiled a bit. "You might go to your grandmother's this weekend."

"Good, then Maggie and I can get away from Sandy."

"Sandy is a nice man. You'll get' to like her," Mom said.

I watched Sandy as she walked down the back porch of that old house. At that moment, she did look like a man to me. I was frightened. How could I be sure that I would grow up to be a lady as Mom had promised? Was it possible that I could grow up to be a man?

WHERE ARE WE GOING?

"Wake up, Maggie!" Mom ordered as we arrived at Jeckler's Shop. Sandy opened the car door for us. Maggie opened the back door for herself and hopped out. As Mom lifted me out, she said, "Sandy, get Maggie's hand."

"Just one second." After locking the car, Sandy reached into the back pocket of her man's dungarees and combed her hair with a little black comb. Mom said, "Sandy, I think you need a haircut.

I thought to myself, *It looks short enough already*, but Sandy said, "Okay, darling...."

We entered the store. Mom took me past the staring crowd to the rear and laid me on my stomach on the floor. As she searched for dresses that would fit me, Maggie ran to me, "Here's the coat I want, Teeny!"

"Okay, try it on," I smiled.

Mom said, "I don't like it. Take it back." Maggie started to cry, but Mom ignored her. She asked, "Like this dress, Teeny?" It was red and green.

"Yes, but...." It didn't matter. She'd buy it no matter how I felt.

Maggie returned the pretty coat, then came back and sat on the floor behind me. I said quietly, "When I became a lady and can walk, I'll write a book, make lots of money, come back here, and buy you that coat."

Mom picked out several items for us then heard at the cash register, "Fifty-three-forty-two, please."

She called Sandy over. "I need more money."

Sandy gave her the extra money, then whispered, "This would be an easy spot."

I overheard this. What were they talking about?

Mom paid the cashier and picked me up with, "C'mon Maggie. It's

9

time to go."

Outside she said, "Do you know that their panties went up to forty-nine cents?"

Sandy asked, "How many come in a pack?"

"Four."

"These prices are ridiculous!" Sandy complained.

On the way home, they stopped at the supermarket, leaving Maggie and me alone in the car.

"Teeny, won't you be glad to go over to Momma's house? She cooks good greens and corn bread, don't you think?" Maggie asked.

I answered, "Yes, I'll be glad to go!"

"Teeny, why did you bite Sandy? She's been so nice to us."

"Never mind about that. I'm still gonna get you that new coat when I'm a lady."

Sandy returned with a bag of groceries. Maggie asked, "Where's Mommy?"

"She'll be right out," Sandy assured us. Then she sat in the car and tried to be friends with me, "Teeny, have you ever been to a football game?"

"No, football's for boys—not girls."

She persisted, "What do you like to do besides watch television?"

"I don't want to be your friend."

She opened her mouth, but Maggie called, "Here's Mom!" And that was that.

When we got home, Mom asked, "What about dinner? I can bake some macaroni and make some greens and corn bread."

Everybody agreed. Sandy took me to Mom's room and turned on the TV. "What would you like to watch?" she asked.

"The Twilight Zone."

She sat next to me, then asked, "Do you know how to play checkers?"

"No."

"Well, I'll teach you."

She brought out the checkerboard and set up the pieces. As she explained the game, I wondered, *Now, how am I supposed to move the pieces*?

Sandy put a pencil in my mouth, "Just push the pieces with this."

I didn't want to play with her, but I was tired of TV.

She won the first game. Halfway through the second game, I started to pick up the pieces with my lips and tongue. Strange...l was having fun with someone I didn't like.

"Time to eat!" Mom called.

Sandy carried me downstairs and laid me on the dining room floor. I watched Maggie set the table. Mom instructed, "The forks are in the drawer under the sink, child." (You see, we usually ate in my bedroom.) Sandy, Mom, and Maggie ate at the table. I ate laying on the floor, with a pillow to comfort my stomach.

"Frances, why didn't you report that your furniture was stolen?" Sandy asked.

"I can't have no cops coming in here. They'd find out about my whole operation," Mom answered.

"Mom, are you a doctor?" Maggie wanted to know.

"What do you mean?" Mom asked.

"You say you 'operate,' like on 'General Hospital,' Maggie explained.

"No, I'm not no doctor. Put the plates in the sink. Come on, Teeny, time for bed."

"Mom, can we watch TV in your room?"

"Yes, I'm goin' out for a little while."

Oh...another three days alone, I thought.

Soon Mom and Sandy were gone and Maggie and I were in front of the TV alone. But I wasn't too frightened this time. She did not lock us in.

We watched and watched TV until Maggie fell asleep. I didn't want to sleep until Mom came back. I was afraid that Maggie would be hurt if Mom was not home when she awakened. But I was just being silly. After all Mom had bought us clothes, lots of food was in the kitchen, and the bedroom door was unlocked. And so I slept.

I awakened early. Mom wasn't home. *Maggie's gonna be upset when she wakes up!* I thought.

But then I heard, "Teeny!" Maggie opened her eyes and said, "Mommy is home! She didn't leave us?" She ran downstairs. Soon she ran back and announced gleefully, "Mom got me that coat I wanted!"

Up the stairs came my mother and Sandy, smiling broadly. Their arms were filled with dresses, coats, underwear, shirts, blouses, socks, and everything!

"Mommy went shopping again last night!" Maggie laughed.

Mom said, "Maggie, go get a comb so I can do you–all hair."

Maggie couldn't find our comb, so Mom said, "Come here so I can dress you. I want you to go to the store."

After my sister was dressed, Mom gave her fifty cents and said, "Go to Trankie's on the corner and buy a comb."

Sandy walked up the stairs, her brogans clomp–clomping all the way. "Frances, I hope nobody saw us."

Mom sucked her teeth, "You're worrying about nuthin'. Sandy approached Mom and tried to kiss her, but Mom pushed her away. Sandy asked, "What's wrong with you?"

"Come in the bathroom. I want t' talk to you." They left.

I was worried about Maggie. She was too young to go to the store all by herself. But soon she banged on the front door. Since the bathroom door was closed, Mom didn't hear her.

"Mom! Maggie's at the door!" I shouted.

Sandy went to let Maggie in. Mom returned to her bedroom with tears in her eyes. "What's wrong, Mom?"

"Nuthin'! Just got some dust in my eyes."

When Maggie and Sandy entered our bedroom, Mom asked, "Where's the comb?"

Maggie shrugged, "I didn't have enough...."

"What? I gave you fifty cents!"

"A man on the corner asked me for change and this is what he gave me. So Trankie said that I didn't have enough." Maggie showed Mom two bright pennies.

"What's wrong with you, givin' away my damn money?" Maggie began crying. "I'm gonna give you something t' cry about!" Mom shouted, grabbing Maggie's arm and dragging her into our bedroom. "Sandy, give me the belt!"

Sandy handed Mom the belt from her dungarees.

"Take off that damn coat!" I heard. Then I could hear the awful belt upon my four–year–old sister's body. Her cries became louder and louder as Mom shouted, "I'm gonna teach you about givin' away my damn money!"

Suddenly, crash! Something had landed on the floor. Maggie had stopped crying. I cringed in that bed.

Sandy ran into our little bedroom and returned with Maggie in her arms. My little sister appeared to be asleep. Sandy put her on the bed very gently, then asked, "Frances, what made you beat this child like that? You're smoking too many of them damn joints." She patted Maggie's face, "This child is unconscious."

I turned myself over and pushed my little sister's face with my chin. "Maggie, Maggie," I cried softly. She didn't move.

Sandy and Mom went into the next room and left us alone.

Finally, slowly, my sister opened her eyes. She looked up at me and put her arms around my neck, crying bitterly.

"Don't cry, Maggie. Just wait 'til I become a lady."

And then there was a loud banging on our front door. Mom ordered, "Go find out who's at the door, Sandy."

Sandy came into Mom's bedroom and looked out the window. She ran back, "Frances, it's the cops!"

Mom grabbed her pocketbook and coat. Sandy got her car keys and coat. Quietly, and without a word to us, they raced down the steps and out the back door.

Finally the banging stopped. The cops did not enter the house.

Maggie laid her head on my shoulder and whispered, "Wish I could go to sleep and never wake up. She beat me, then she picked me up high over her head, then she threw me on the floor. She's not Mommy anymore, Teeny. You are."

Her eyes began to close. But she had a great big hickey on

her forehead. Momma, had warned us not to let a child who had fallen go to sleep right away because the child might not wake up. I was frightened.

"Stay awake, Maggie. You remember what Momma said. Get up, walk around now. You can't sleep!"

Slowly she got up. "My leg's hurtin'."

"Well, just stand there then."

"Please don't be so mean, Teeny. Let me lay down."

"You got to remember what Momma said."

"Humph! If I could carry you, we'd run away from home."

"No need for that, we're goin' to Momma's."

"When? I'm sleepy now."

"Maggie, you lay down, and I'll bite you good!"

She didn't cry. "I'm sleepy."

How could I, laying in a bed, keep my sister awake? Then I remembered something I'd seen Mom do to a drunken man who'd visited the house. And so I said, "Tell you what. Go get some ice from the fridge and put It on y'r head. You'll feel better, I promise. Then, I'll let you go to sleep."

Maggie started down the hall. I heard a crash. *Oh God, she fell down!*

"Maggie! Maggie!" I shouted. There was no answer. How could I get to her? How could I help her?

I turned on my back and slid to the edge of the bed. Slowly I plopped to the floor. Ouch! my butt. The first splinter on my butt. Never mind. I had to move the trunk of my body toward the door, with splinters cutting my skin all the way. I turned over, hoping to move faster on my back, but the splinters pulled my hair and pierced my scalp. I had to turn over again and move on my stomach.

Finally I reached Maggie, who laid on the hallway floor.

"Maggie, Maggie, why didn't you answer me?"

"I heard you, but I was sleepy...."

"Get up and go get that ice or else I'm gonna beat you!"

"How, Teeny? You can't even hold a belt."

"I got here, didn't I? If you don't get up right now, you'll find out how!"

I gave her one mean look, then guarded the stairs as she went down. She returned with ice in her bare hands.

"You should have put it in a dishrag or something," I suggested.

"I didn't know about that, Teeny."

"There's an old sock in the bathroom hamper. Put the ice in it, then put it on your head."

She did so. I ordered, "Hold it up now on your head!"

Maggie bawled, "This ice is too cold. I want to go to sleep.

"Ice is suppos' t' be cold. Stay awake!"

"Come on, Teeny. I'll help you off this floor. It must hurt down there."

"Never mind about that. Just you stand right here with that ice on y'r head, Maggie!"

We stayed in that hallway 'til it got dark.

The ice in that sock melted. The hickey on Maggie's forehead had gone down just a bit. "Put that sock in the sink, Maggie."

I slid across the floor with all those splinter, and Maggie helped me back into bed. "Can I go to sleep now, Teeny?"

"I guess so." But I was still scared. And so I watched Maggie asleep for hours, just to make sure that she was still breathing.

Then I heard, "Sandy, go see if the cops took th' kids."

"Teeny," Sandy called.

I wouldn't answer. I didn't like her.

She ran upstairs. "Why didn't you answer me, Teeny?"

"Because I didn't want to!"

"The cops been here?"

"Nobody came in. Why don't you think about Maggie? She still got that big hickey on her forehead."

"How'd she get a hickey from a strap?"

"Mom threw her on the floor. Didn't you know?"

"No, and I left her like that?" Concern was in Sandy's eyes. She sat down, picked up Maggie, and rocked her to and fro.

We looked up. There was Mom, listening all the while. She said, "Put that damn girl down, Sandy. There's nuthin' wrong with her."

"Come see this big hickey on her head, Frances."

"I don't give a damn. Start packing."

I asked, "Mom, where we goin'?"

"You're not goin' anywhere. Just me an' Sandy. We have to go away for a few days."

"It's two o'clock in the morning, Frances. Let's wait 'til morning," Sandy pleaded.

Mom sniffed, "Oh sure—an' let the cops get us."

Sandy laid Maggie on the bed and said, "I got a good idea." She went to the phone and called the police station. She whispered into the phone, "I got a hot tip for you. Heard you were lookin' for Frances Tate and Sandy Jones. Well, I seen them on Sixty–third an' Haverford. You know, The Speakeasy."

I could hear the cop answer, "Why you telling us this, miss?"

"Because both them bulldaggers jumped me one night. When they were through, they stole my whole welfare money." She slammed down the phone.

"That's the oldest trick in the book. This is the first place they gonna look," Mom said.

"I don't think so. We'll be on guard. After all I can't leave Maggie and Teeny like this."

Mom snapped back, "Why should you care? They're not your fuckin' kids. They'se mine, damnit!"

Tears rolled down my face.

Sandy was angry, "Somebody got to care. You with your red, green, and gold joints don't. She picked up Maggie and put her in our room. Mom looked at me, "What the hell you crying about? Maybe you want what I gave Maggie."

Sandy returned with, "Stop it, Frances! Now you've gone too far."

She picked me up, took me into our bedroom and laid me next to Maggie. She kissed me and whispered, "Let me talk to your mother. Watch out for Maggie and call me if she needs anything." She closed the door halfway and returned to Mom. I heard a lot of arguing.

"You're getting too damn close to my kids, Sandy!" There was a loud slap. My mother cried and Sandy snarled, "How does it feel to get slapped around, Frances?"

Mom ran down the stairs. When she ran back up, as she passed, I could see a great big butcher knife in her hand. I shivered as she yelled, "I'm going to cut your God–damn throat Sandy! No mother fucker is going to put their hands on me."

Then there was a sound of somebody being choked. At that moment, Maggie began to vomit in bed.

"Sandy, Sandy!" I shouted, "Maggie is throwing up."

Sandy rushed in, threw the butcher knife over the bed, and rushed Maggie to the bathroom.

"Frances, come see about your child, she's sick!"

I watched through the door as Mom lifted the pillow from her face. She was coughing. She made her way out into the bathroom and said hoarsely, "There's nothing wrong with her. She's just cutting up."

"She can't pretend to throw up, Frances. Hand me that towel." Sandy washed Maggie, carried her in and laid her on our other twin bed. She put me there too so that she could remove the sheet on which Maggie had vomited.

Then Sandy whispered, "Teeny, try to sleep now. Maggie will be all right, and I won't leave you two alone tonight."

She walked into Mom's bedroom and I could hear her say, "Stop the shit, Frances, and let's get to bed."

I went to sleep without worry.

The next morning Maggie awakened me with, "My head hurts, Teeny."

"Go tell Sandy; maybe she'll give you an aspirin." Maggie did so.

Mom appeared and said, "What kinda cereal you want, Teeny?"

"Cornflakes, with lotsa sugar." She disappeared, saying nothing.

"Somebody's at the door!" Sandy shouted.

"You better look out first. It may be th' cops!" Mom said.

"It's Mr. Miletti."

I was happy. That insurance man always had lots of paper and pencils for Maggie. But since I last saw him, I'd learned to do many more things with my mouth. I couldn't wait to see what he had because I'd made a secret bet with myself that I could write, too.

Mom said, "C'mon up, Sal!"

The insurance man ran up the stairs and into Mom's bedroom.

Sandy and Maggie came to me.

"Want to watch TV, Teeny?" Sandy asked.

"Yeah," I answered. She carried me into Mom's bedroom while Maggie followed. Mr. Miletti said to my little sister, "Here, squirt. Here's some paper and pencils, just for you." As usual he rubbed the top of my head gently and asked, "How you doin', Teeny?"

"Fine. Where's my paper and pencils?" I pouted with a smile.

He jumped with amazement. "When did you start writing, smarty pants?"

I said, trembling, "Right now." I remembered drawing pictures with my foot. But they didn't come out well because I couldn't see as I drew. Now, quietly, I asked, "Sandy, how does my name go?"

Sandy took one of Mr. Miletti's big drawing pads, sat next to me, and very slowly, she wrote in big print, "Celestine Tate."

Then she put the pencil in my mouth. Everyone was silent as I tried to copy exactly what Sandy had written with that pencil in my mouth.

When I was through, I looked up. My eyes met Mr. Miletti's and I wondered, *Why does Mr. Miletti look so sad now? He's always telling jokes.*

"I know it's bad now, Mr. Miletti, but I'll get better. Sandy, will you help me practice?"

"It's not too bad, Teeny...." he answered, then turned around. Sandy said, "Yup, you got a lot of work t' do, Teeny!"

I grinned, looking at all that paper I had to practice on. But then I stopped, for Mom said, "Humph! Those damn kids always got t' be the center of attention!"

Mr. Miletti turned around and asked, "Got the insurance, Frances?"

"Come in the bathroom, and we'll talk about it," Mom answered. They left.

Sandy looked at Maggie, who'd been scribbling on the floor all the while. "Need any help, Maggie?"

"Nope," my sister said cheerfully.

Mom called from the bathroom, "Come here, Sandy." Sandy left.

Maggie climbed on the bed and together, we scribbled our letters, numbers, and some funny pictures of Mr. Miletti.

Sandy returned, "You'll have to go in your own room now."

"What about watching TV?" I asked.

"I'll take it in there."

"How can you carry that big set, Sandy?"

"Sandy's as strong as a man!" Maggie giggled.

Soon my sister and I were watching TV from our twin bed. Mom left the bathroom and quietly entered her bedroom. Mr. Miletti followed her. Strange, after he had entered her bedroom, she had locked the door.

Sandy slumped out of the bathroom and stomped down the stairs. "I got to see about the car, Teeny. I'll be back in a little while." Then she ran down the stairs and slammed the door.

Maggie and I remained glued to the TV that Sunday morning; after all it was a Shirley Temple movie. Maggie kept humming, but I could hear everything, even Mom's door unlocking. I turned my head slightly. There was Mr. Miletti coming down the hall with no clothes on. But my mother was not married to Mr. Miletti. She couldn't be because he wasn't even our color. So it was not funny to me that he had no clothes on.

When he entered the bathroom, I whispered quickly, "Maggie, I'm cold. Close the hall door."

"I'm not cold, but okay...." she answered, closing the door.

"Turn up the TV. I can't hear it too good," I said,

"What! Momma says you hear like a watchdog, Teeny, an' we been hearing okay so far. But, oh, well...," and she turned up the TV.

So Maggie did not see or hear Mr. Miletti return to Mom's bedroom. But I heard Mom's door unlock. I heard Mom say, "See you next week, Sal."

"Okay, Frances. Kiss the kids goodbye for me."

I looked at all those lovely pencils and paper with sadness.

Mom opened our bedroom door and said, "You all finished y'r cornflakes yet?"

Before Maggie could answer, I said, "Maggie, go get my pot. I have to pee." Maggie left.

"Mom, why didn't Mr. Miletti have any clothes on?"

"He wanted to take a bath," she answered nonchalantly, collecting our empty bowls.

Maggie returned. I turned over, and she put the pot under me. I peed quickly, thinking, *Mr. Miletti sure takes a fast bath.*

My sister took the pot back to the bathroom. "Be careful you don't spill none," Mom warned. The downstairs door slammed. "That you Sandy?" she asked.

"Yes, you took care of that insurance money, Frances?"

"Yeah, he'll hold off for another month."

Sandy raced up the stairs in those broghan shoes. Mom reached out to her, but got, "Get away from me!"

"I was only lookin' out for all of us, Sandy," Mom pleaded.

"You had the insurance money, but no, you had to spend it on those joints," Sandy grumbled. Then she looked at me, laying in that bed. Something in my face made her ask, "What's wrong, Teeny? Did she say something mean to you?"

"Ain't nuthin' wrong with me. You actin' like you're my father or something...."

Maggie turned her eyes from the TV and laughed, "Sure she could be our father. She can lift the TV good enough." Her eyes returned to Shirley Temple.

Mom said, "Come in our bedroom, Sandy. I got to talk to you."

But Sandy ordered, "No. Go take off that nightgown and get on some clothes, Frances."

So Mom left alone, while Sandy sat with me. She said sadly, "I don't know why you don't like me; you even bit me. But I love you and Maggie, Teeny."

I turned away from her and watched my beautiful mother put on one of those nice checkered dresses with the white collar and cuffs. She was just putting her foot into a nylon stocking when Bang! Bang! Bang! on the front door.

"Who th' hell's that, Sandy?" Mom yelled running into our room. Sandy sped to the front window. "It's th' cops!" She raced to our toy room window and screeched, "They're at th' back door, too! We can't get out no way!"

Maggie saw the fear on Mom and Sandy's faces. She ran and grabbed Mom, "Who's banging, Mommy? Is somebody gonna kill us?"

My mother shoved her to the floor, "Get outta th' way!"

Sandy picked up Maggie, but my little sister scrambled away from her and into my bed. She put her arms around my neck tightly, "Teeny, what's wrong? I'm scared!"

For the first time, I had no answer for her. "Just be quiet 'fore the cops hear you."

The banging continued. Mom panted, "Let's go to the roof and hope that they leave." She turned to us, "If they get in here, you better not say anything about where we're at."

She and Sandy raced up the stairs silently, without another word.

My little sister and I clung together as that awful banging and banging continued. Finally the front door crashed open!

"Upstairs! They must still be here. Their car is still out back," a man said.

Then we could see several cops rush through the hallway into Mom's room. They looked like those who raided the Mafia on "The Untouchables."

"They're not in here! You go that way," the biggest cop yelled to a couple more cops.

Maggie couldn't control her crying anymore and bawled out loud.

"Somebody's in the other room!" we heard. And what seemed like a dozen cops rushed into our little bedroom, with their guns fully drawn.

"No!" Maggie screamed, clutching my neck.

"Please, please don't shoot us!" I cried out.

They were aghast. "What the hell do we have here?" said the biggest cop with the bright red hair. "Put th' damn guns away, fellas."

Another big cop asked, "Okay, where's y'r mother and that dyke, kid?"

"Gee, I...I don't know where they went. They been gone all night," I sobbed.

The biggest cop looked at a smaller one and said, "You mean those bitches left these kids alone all night?"

The latter said, "No...she's lying." He turned to me and said "You know where they are. Tell us, NOW!"

Maggie sobbed. I whispered, "Be quiet." My brain raced wildly. Then, with eyes opened wide and innocent, I said, "I don't know what you mean. We're here by ourselves all the time."

"Who feeds you?"

"Mom always feeds us before she leaves...."

A third cop, the one with blonde hair said, "We can't leave these kids here. Those women know we're after 'em, so they won't come back now."

The big cop said to us, "Well, kids, get up an' get y'r clothes on...."

Slowly, Maggie slid off my back. I was exposed.

The cops yelped, "Oh, God, she's crippled!"

The blonde one hissed, "And they left her...."

An older one came close and asked softly, "Who dresses you when your Mom's not here?"

"I do," little Maggie whispered.

I took a deep breath, then suggested, "If you all leave for awhile, we can get our clothes on." They left.

Remembering Mom and Sandy shivering on the roof, I said, "Come on, Maggie. If we hurry, they might give us something nice to eat." I didn't mention my fear of being shot by those cops. Maggie didn't pay attention to the news the way I did, so she didn't know that a bunch of cops had shot a boy in the Five and Ten just last night.

She pulled on her little panties, shirt, and dress. Then she trotted over with my clothes and helped me as I wiggled into them.

I whispered, "Don't say one word to those to those cops about nuthin'. You don't know nuthin', about nobody, no way no how, y' hear me? Else they'll take Mom and Sandy to jail, and we'll never see 'em, ever again."

"Why are the cops after 'em, Teeny? What did they do?"

"I don't know, but if we keep our mouths shut and just listen, we'll find out from the cops."

"Okay, Teeny," she nodded. Then she added sadly, "Those are real guns they got, ain't they?"

"Yeah, just remember that, and keep quiet."

"Are you dressed yet?" came from the hallway.

"Yes," I answered. Maggie got our coats from Mom's room. She looked at her pretty new coat rejectedly.

The big cop carried me out and laid me on the floor of the police wagon. Fortunately it was too early that Sunday morning for our neighbors to see. Maggie sat next to the big cop and said nothing.

It was a long bumpy ride to the police station. I had a hard time keeping my mouth out of the dirt on the floor. I felt as though I was the rug that should have covered that filthy floor.

At last we were in the police station. The cop at the desk looked up and asked in surprise, "Who are they?"

"Two abandoned ones from the Tate–Jones robbery. They were at the house alone," said the big cop.

"Why are you carrying her? Is she sick?"

"No, she's crippled."

There he goes with that word again. Since we were in the house all alone most of the time, I'd never heard it before. And I couldn't wait to ask my father what it meant.

A heavy–set lady cop came out of one of the offices and picked me up, took Maggie by the hand, and walked us down a long hall to a cell. Then she laid me on a cot and helped me take my coat off. She said that she was going off duty and there would be another lady cop along to help us, and for us not to be afraid.

Soon it was dinner time. This big white cop with red hair came into the cell and asked Maggie and me if we were hungry.

Maggie anxiously said, "Yes."

So the cop came back soon with hamburgers and cold French fries.

As Maggie was eating, tears began to slowly run from her eyes, and then I knew it was going to be a hard, cold night.

GOING TO GRANDMA'S

It was a hard, cold night, as I remember. My only warmth was Maggie's body laying on my back. I was really scared. Would they take Maggie away from me? She didn't know anything about Mom being wanted by the police, so when she'd wake up and learn that Mom was never coming back, she'd be terrified. I thought *I hope daytime comes quickly because I've got to reach Momma as soon as possible.* Maggie was very happy about going to Momma's, although she loved Mom. As for me, I hoped I'd never see Mom again.

I looked through the bars of that cell and saw an old fat lady mopping the floor of the hallway. She looked over and said to me, "What are you doing here? What's wrong with you?"

I said quietly, "There's nuthin' wrong with me." Suddenly a big iron door slammed. A cop was standing at the cell.

"Do you have to go the bathroom, kid?"

Maggie woke up. She looked confused, but we both nodded, "Yes."

He opened the cell door and let Maggie out. "Turn down the hall, on the right is the bathroom."

I said, "Turn toward the wall, Maggie, that's the right side."

The cop wrinkled his whole face, "An' how do you go to the bathroom?"

"The other cops didn't give us time to bring my pot."

He scratched his head, "Wait a minute kid. I'll find something for you."

Soon he was back with a small wash basin. He entered the cell and asked, "What should I do now?"

"Never mind, Mister. When my sister comes back from the bathroom, she'll help me go."

He shook his head, "No, I'll do it. She doesn't feel well, remember."

Since I was lying on the cot, I could hardly see his face. It was so high above his fat stomach. He bent down, turned me on my stomach and pulled down my panties. Then he put me on the basin and let me pee.

I knew that everything was all right. He was just trying to help me.

When I was through, he removed the basin, turned me flat on my back and pulled my legs apart. Then he stuck his big, dirty, hard finger inside me.

I didn't know what was going on. I jumped, then said, "Please don't do that, Mister!" I couldn't figure out why he would do such a thing. All I knew was that I felt insulted, both physically and mentally.

And then we heard Maggie skip down the hall. Quickly, the cop pulled out his finger and restored my panties. He picked up the basin and said, "Get back in here, kid." Maggie entered quietly. That cop slammed out of the cell.

I wanted to cry but couldn't. I had enough to explain to Maggie without confusing her with my tears. So...I said, "Come here, Maggie. Put your head on my face so I can tell if you got a fever."

She lay with her face next to mine. Her face was burning. I looked around that tiny cell and thought, *No wonder she's got a fever. Even though it's so cold, there's no window in here. I can't even tell if it's day or night.*

Someone else walked toward us. He stopped at our cell. It was another cop, but he was different. He was our color. He opened the cell door, came in, and sat on a stool next to our cot. He said to Maggie, "Why are you shivering like that? Are you cold?"

I wanted to tell him what the other cop had done to me, but I was afraid he wouldn't believe me. Besides Maggie couldn't learn of this.

Maggie answered, "I sure am. It's freezing in here."

"I saw, on TV, they let criminals in prison have one phone call."

He laughed, "Who you got in mind, baby?"

"Our Momma. She would come and get us outta here."

"What's your Momma's name and phone number?"

"All I know is her name is Momma Tate."

"What about her first name, hon?"

Maggie said, "She's our grandma, so her name's Momma. Momma, of course."

He said with a sigh, "I'll see what I can do," then he stamped out whispering something about "treating homeless kids like they were crooks."

Maggie asked hoarsely, "Teeny, what does he mean by that?"

"I think he's talking about orphans, like in the Shirley Temple movie we were watching yesterday."

"But Teeny, Shirley Temple didn't go to jail for being an orphan! You're wrong!"

"No, I'm not, Maggie; TV is only pretend while we are really in jail."

And so we laid down and looked at those ugly iron bars.

Finally, that nice cop came back. "I just got finished talkin' to y'r Momma and she said that she'll send y'r daddy to get you soon as he gets home from work."

Tears filled our eyes. We cried, "Gee thanks, Mister!"

"It's nuthin', sweethearts," he said, and he left.

Maggie asked, "Teeny, if you didn't know Momma's number, how did that cop get it?"

"Oh, Maggie, cops can find anybody they want." (But I remembered sadly the cops battering down our door. They probably had a big file on Mom and Sandy, just like Elliot Ness always had on criminals.) And so I continued, "Just forget cops. Don't you want something to eat?"

"No ... I'm too sleepy."

I thought, *Oh, she really must be sick if she don't want to eat.*

My little sister quietly crawled on my back and went to sleep. I laid and stared at those ugly bars. What was the big difference, being locked in by Mom at home or being locked in jail? Perry Mason always defended people who were charged with some crime. What was I being charged with? I couldn't move, much less rob a store, like Mom and Sandy could.

And then my father's voice came through my thoughts. I shook my back, "Maggie! Maggie! Daddy's here. Get y'r coat!"

Maggie opened her eyes and smiled, "We're going to Momma's now?"

The cop who had brought me that basin came in with Daddy, who said, "Hi, kids. How long you been in this jail?" He scooped up Maggie and gave her a big kiss. "You feel so hot, Maggie. Are you sick?"

I said, "All night long she's had a fever in this freezing cold place."

Daddy bent over, hugged and kissed me, and asked, "They didn't even give you a blanket?" He rose, helped Maggie put on her coat and buttoned it. Since they hadn't taken away my coat, he simply picked me up and shouted, "Let's get the hell outta this dirty jail! Momma's worried sick about you two!"

That was the only time I ever heard my father curse.

The big cop said, "Ya gotta sign 'em out, Mr. Tate."

Dad fumed, "Sure, like they're on probation, huh?"

The cop said, "Oh, never mind that. Have you seen your wife and that dyke she hangs out with?"

"No, I ain't seen neither one in a long time."

Soon we were on a bus. It was the first time I'd been on a bus. Daddy had to give Maggie the money to put in the fare box because he was holding me. Everyone stared as he didn't fall as that bus lurched forward, then backward, for he carried me with one hand and held onto Maggie with the other.

We reached the very back of that bus, but none of those staring riders got up and gave Daddy a seat. "Hold tight to the bar, Maggie," he said as he held on in the middle of the aisle.

"Ouch!" I cried as my head banged on the bar.

Daddy turned and twisted to protect me as several passengers laughed like we were "The Three Stooges."

It was a long, tiresome ride. My daddy's arms must have hurt terribly. But finally we struggled down the steps of that bus. After a short walk, he said, "Oh, three flights of stairs to go. Momma has to live on the third floor of this place."

Maggie held the door as we entered the apartment building. There were many huge four–letter words scrawled in bright paint on those chipped walls. Maggie slammed the front door.

Suddenly a crowd of kids ran down the stairs, crying "Teeny and Maggie are here! Momma! It's Teeny and Maggie!"

Seven dirty black faces stared at me. How did all these kids know Maggie and me? Who were they?"

I looked at Daddy. He smiled, "These are all your cousins, Teeny."

As the kids yelled, I asked, "How come they know me and Maggie, Daddy? We never seen any of them before."

"They live with your Aunt Anita on Franklin Street. It's a shame your mother brought you to Momma's so few times that you never got to meet them when they visited."

Maggie kept giggling as she ran up the stairs with our new–found family. These kids kept turning around to smile at me in my Daddy's arms.

And then I heard, "J.C., is that you? You got the kids?"

"Yes, Momma, we're all here."

We entered Momma's apartment. Momma walked up and gave me one of her real big sloppy kisses.

"J.C., help Teeny take off her coat. She must've been cold out there."

Since Maggie had seven little cousins to help her with her coat, I was only worried about her fever. But Momma would take care of her.

Soon we were drinking Momma's homemade hot chocolate. (Oh, yes, everything Momma served was homemade.) I lay on her kitchen floor and watched the bugs march through the cracks in the woodwork. The room was filled with the aroma of Momma's cooking. I knew that I was going to have a good meal.

Daddy said, "Teeny, I want you to meet your cousins." The kids, who ranged in age from two to twelve years, smiled past me. "Here's Lloyd, Rose, Rusty, Hank, Adrian, Freddy, and Bertha–Mae."

Momma chased them with, "Go wash y'r hands now, it's time t' eat!" I watched the splashy confusion in the nearby bathroom while Momma washed my face and scrubbed my teeth with a damp, soapy cloth. As usual I didn't bother to ask her to rinse the soap out of my mouth.

Momma ordered, "Adrian, Rose—come eat at this table!"

My eldest cousins hurried out of the bathroom, drying their hands quickly on their dresses. I laid on the floor and watched the speed with which they obeyed Momma.

Momma plopped down next to me. Her body hung over the side of the small kitchen chair, and I wondered how that chair could hold her. She brought me down to earth with, "Teeny, you want greens or cabbage t'nite?"

"The greens got hamhocks in 'em, Momma?"

"What other way is there to cook 'em?"

I smiled, "Well, the greens, Momma."

I watched my cousins, then my grandmother, and felt almost safe. But the heat next to that hot stove was unbearable. Eventually I got up enough nerve to wiggle away a bit.

Momma looked at me. "Where you goin'?"

"Oh, just away from the stove. Any closer an' I'll be a part of the dinner."

Momma and my cousins laughed.

I continued, "Momma, when did you move out of the other house?"

"What other house, Teeny?"

"The house with the green porch and the big round bed where you read the Bible to me? I'll never forget the Twenty–third Psalm."

"That's y'r Aunt Silvia's house, child, not mine! I've lived in this tiny apartment for twenty years."

She reached over and got my plate, which Adrian had filled with greens, rice, and oh–some–wonderful fried chicken. (That fried chicken was so good, Momma could've put the chicken kings out of business.) Momma laid the plate on the floor as my cousins sat around the table.

"Lloyd, it's your turn to say grace," Momma said quietly.

Everyone but me folded their hands. I bowed my head with my family as Lloyd hurried through, "Thank You for this food. Amen," and everybody dug in.

My cousins ate, but each in turn stopped and watched me as I picked up my food with my mouth. Then each turned back to his meal and ate a bit more slowly. I thought the only one who didn't interrupt her feast was Maggie.

Daddy said, "You all stop staring at Teeny an' eat your dinner!"

Soon everyone rose and placed his or her plate in the sink. Maggie followed the rest, then came over and took my empty plate from the floor with a contented smile. No words were needed between us.

Daddy picked me up from the floor, took me into Momma's bedroom, and laid me on her large, lumpy bed. He sat beside me and watched as I kept moving around. The springs in that mattress stuck me no matter where I moved.

"What're you moving around like that for, Teeny?"

"Oh, I'm just thinking how much better it is here than in that jail, Daddy."

He sighed, then asked, "You gonna tell me why the cops are lookin' fa y'r mother?"

I thought quickly, remembering Mom's stern orders; "Don't tell anybody a damn thing, Teeny, else I'll break y'r ass!" Besides Daddy still loved Mom too much to believe the worst of her. And so I opened my eyes wide and said, "Gee, Daddy, how 'm I suppos' t' know?"

My dad just sat and held me. The mattress didn't hurt. Finally I fell asleep.

I awakened to silence. Maggie and my cousins must have been asleep in the living room. I heard Momma and Dad in the kitchen.

"J.C., what happened to Frances? Why were those babies in jail?"

"I don't know for sure, Momma. I got a feeling Teeny knows, but she's not ready t' tell me."

"How can she know, J.C.? She's a smart girl, but she's only six, remember? She even asked me when did I move here. She didn't even know we always met at Silvia's house."

"Frances is so involved with those joints and those women, she doesn't have time to take those kids anywhere. It's a miracle she brought 'em to Silvia's."

"So, what we gonna do with them? I don't have enough room here for two more kids. Where they gonna sleep? I can send Maggie to school, but who's gonna watch Teeny when I go to work on the farm?"

"I'll get a baby-sitter for her. She's not much trouble."

"J.C., how you gonna pay a baby sitter? We barely got enough for food and rent every week. If they didn't let me bring home food from th' farm, we'd starve."

"Well, Momma, what can I do, give 'em up for adoption? Nobody wants black kids anyway, an' who would love Teeny?"

I shuddered in the bed and felt the tears on my cheeks. Then Momma pulled me from the edge of the cliff with, "Shut y'r mouth, J.C. I'd never give those kids up for adoption."

There was silence. I waited. I heard Daddy jump from his chair and say, "What about the Welfare? They pay for kids who need babysitters, don't they? Besides we got Rose an' all the others on Welfare, why not Teeny and Maggie?"

"The Welfare is not going to go for two more kids in this one—bedroom apartment. They don't want t' give us money for the seven we already got here."

"Mom, don't you know yet when Anita's gonna get her kids?"

"Well, she said she'd come for 'em last month, but she never showed up. She didn't even call Aunt Ethel t' let me know where she was."

"It's your fault, Momma. You always, I mean always, Momma, lovin' too much all those kids and lettin' 'em take advantage of you."

"I love all my kids an' grandkids, and I'll take care of them as long as they need me. I don't think Anita will be that much longer without her kids."

"But you've been sayin' that for the last three months, Momma. It was much easier when Daddy was alive, but it's too much for us to handle all these kids all by ourselves now."

"Well, the only thing for us to do is to talk to the social worker an' figure out how we'll take care of Maggie, an' especially Teeny."

The sound of church music came from Momma's small kitchen radio. Then came Maggie's voice, "Momma, I gotta go to the bathroom. Is Teeny still sleepin'?"

My grandmother answered, "Yeah, she ate enough chicken. Must've been starved. By the way, Maggie, don't you have any slippers?"

"Sure, Mommy bought me three pairs when she an' Sandy bought us all those clothes an' my new coat yesterday. But all our stuff's home. The cops wouldn't let us take 'em."

I knew what Maggie would blab next, so I yelled, "Maggie! Maggie! Would you help me turn over?"

"Okay, Teeny, I'm comin'. Just let me go pee."

Momma said, "J.C., where would Frances get all that money to buy all those clothes at one time, especially with her habit?"

Daddy whispered, "Gee...Maggie's probably exaggeratin', as usual...."

Maggie entered the bedroom, and I whispered quickly, "Remember, Mom said t' shut up 'bout all those clothes an' stuff, or else!"

Maggie rubbed her sleep–filled eyes. "Okay, Teeny. Okay," and she left.

Momma came in. "Why didn't Maggie turn you over as you asked?" As Momma turned me over, I closed my eyes and forgot to thank her. She returned to my father and said, "I wonder what that was all about?" She returned quickly to the bedroom, but my eyes were shut tight. "Guess she's gone back to sleep, J.C.."

"Yeah, guess so." There was no more conversation.

I listened to that holy music for what seemed like hours until Momma slid into bed next to me and began to snore. Then I spent the night listening to her snore.

Early the next morning, I heard Rose say, "That's my shirt! You can't wear it!"

Momma stopped the squabble. "Come into the shed. I'll get you a shirt."

I wondered why they were up so early. Maggie ran in, "Momma's takin' me to a real school today! All our new cousins go there. Isn't that wonderful?"

"That's great, Maggie. You be good now, and remember to keep y'r mouth shut; about new clothes, cops, Sandy, anything about Mom."

My sister left, only a bit deflated. Momma entered and I asked, "Who's gonna stay here while you take Maggie and the others t' school?"

Your daddy doesn't have to go to work 'til three o'clock, so he'll be with you 'til I get back." She bent down and kissed me, "It'll be alright; we'll work it out, Teeny."

Soon everyone left for school. I remember the look of excitement on Maggie's face as she waved goodbye to me.

Daddy watched me as the others left. Then he scooped me from the bed with, "Grits or oatmeal for breakfast, Teeny?"

"Oatmeal, Daddy! What did Maggie have?"

"The kids get free breakfast in school. That's when Momma rushes 'em out early."

Daddy laid me on the kitchen floor and hummed as he stirred our breakfast. He stopped humming and asked, "Do you know anything interesting you'd like to talk about?"

"Yes, Daddy. I'd like to talk about how mean that big cop was to me when I was in jail."

"What? What did he say to you, Teeny?"

"When Maggie went to the bathroom, he got a basin for me an'...an'...."

"An' what, Teeny? You know you can tell me."

"Well, um...after he took me off the pail, he turned me over an' um...well, um.. he stuck his finger, um...um...."

"What!"

"He stuck his finger in me! He hurt me, Daddy!"

My father picked me up from the floor and hugged me, "Oh, God, I'm gonna kill him! Tell me, was he our color or white?"

"No, he wasn't our color; the one our color was nice. He called Momma, Daddy."

There was a bubble from the stove. "Oh, I burned th' oatmeal." Dad turned off the stove and huffed, "We'll eat later, Teeny. Let's get dressed. We got some business to take care of."

It was easy for Maggie to dress me, with my legs folded backwards. She'd done it since she was three. But it was quite difficult for my inexperienced father. He fumbled nervously, muttering to himself, but finally, I was all bundled up.

The trolley ride seemed swifter today. We had a seat and something on our minds besides the stares of the ignorant.

Soon my father marched up the stairs of the Police Station. "Do we have to go in there again, Daddy?"

"Yes," was his grim answer.

He entered and went straight to the captain's desk. "One of your officer's assaulted my daughter yesterday."

The captain answered indifferently, "Which one was it—if any?"
"Never mind, I'll find him myself."

As Dad marched down the hall, three other officers walked behind him. He pushed me up near his shoulder. I turned my head, and saw that cop!

"He's the cop, the one that hurt me, Daddy!"

Quickly Daddy laid me on a bench and ran toward that cop. One of the cops behind us shouted, "Stop nigger—or we'll shoot y'r ass!"

Daddy kept going. He reached that cop and grabbed him by the throat. The other cops had their guns drawn, but couldn't shoot because Dad was too close to that bad cop. Soon Dad was punching that cop on the Police Station floor. I was hollering from the bench, "Get 'im, Dad! Get 'im!"

Soon a pile of cops rushed up and separated my Daddy from that cop. That lousy cop pulled himself from the floor and turned around. He had a black eye!

I yelled, "Momma always say, 'God don't like ugly!'"

"Niggers 'r always tryin' t' take the law into their own hands!" one cop shouted. "They never know when they've had enough and lost."

"Yeah, well what we gonna do when nobody even believes what he did to my helpless little girl?" Dad shouted.

"Get y'r kid, boy. We're lockin' you up for assault on an officer," another cop answered.

"Arrest that cop for assaulting my child!" Daddy cried as he grabbed me and was forced into a cell.

The captain came down the corridor and into the cell with us. He said, "Sit down, Mr. Tate."

Daddy held me as we sat on the cot. The Captain continued, "You have assaulted a police officer, and I am supposed to read you your rights."

"You better be reading that cop his rights, too!" Dad yelled.

"But no one was seriously hurt, so we are willing to forget the whole thing. After all, an assault on an officer is from two to five years in prison. I don't think that is what you're looking for, Mr. Tate."

"Please, Daddy, I'm ready to go home now. Please?" I pleaded.

"I'll forget about everything, but only because I got to take care of my kids now. Otherwise five years wouldn't mean nuthin' t' me if I could tell the world about that cruel cop." Tears rolled down my Daddy's face.

"Open the door and let us out," said the Captain. Daddy picked me up and soon we climbed mournfully onto the trolley once again.

After a long, silent ride, we entered our dingy apartment building. As we started up the stairs, a woman cussed, "Where you been all God-damn day, nigger?"

A man answered, "I had t' work late, sweetheart."

"Don't talk that shit t' me. You promised not t'see her no more!"

"I was workin', honest!"

Dad rushed back down the stairs as, there in the hallway stood a fat woman with a gun. "I'm gonna kill you this time, nigger! Did you hear what I said? I'm gonna kill you this time, nigger!"

Quickly Dad ducked behind the door as the man raced down the stairs.

But that man wasn't fast enough. "Bang!" "Bang!" and on the third "Bang!" the man tumbled all the way down the stairs. The woman slammed into her second floor apartment.

Daddy jumped quickly over the body of that bleeding man and raced up the stairs into Momma's apartment.

I dug my head into my father's chest to block out the violence and cruelty I had experienced in just twenty–four hours. I sobbed at the tricks I'd had to play on my own precious family. Was this what life would be like "when I was a lady?"

As I tried to get the sight of that bleeding man sprawled in the hallway out of my mind, my father hugged me. So gently, he placed me on Momma's bed and removed my coat. Then he returned me to the kitchen and laid me on my blanket, which was in it's usual place near that warm stove. This time the heat was consoling.

Daddy tried to look happy. "Well, we burned th' oatmeal; how 'bout some eggs'n ketchup, Teeny?"

I nodded, "Yes." He hummed again, but so vigorously that he burned the eggs, too. But never mind, at last we had something to eat, and we were together.

As he sat on the floor next to me with our burned breakfast, Dad said, "You ain't never gonna be hurt by no cop, no more, no way. So please Teeny try not to think of this whole business, though I know it's not possible for you to forget it."

"Daddy, what about the man downstairs? Is he dead?"

"I dunno; just eat y'r breakfast, hon."

Then came the cops up the stairs. "Who lives in 3 A?"

"The Tates, with all them kids," said Miss Hippo, the lady next door to us.

Daddy only had to give me a look as he waited. Finally came the knock on our door. "There was a man killed downstairs, boy. You hear or see anything?" the white cop asked.

"No, I didn't hear nuthin'. Just get away from my damn door!" Dad answered. "An' stop callin' me 'boy'!" he added.

After a few curses, the cops left. I asked, "Whatever happened to the lady that shot him, Daddy?"

"She's probably at the train station with a shoppin' bag, lookin' innocent. Since all colored folk look the same to them, they'll never catch her. They probably don't even care."

He put our breakfast dishes in the sink and turned on the radio. Finally came the laughter and the giggling and the stamping up the stairs of Maggie and my seven cousins. I was so relieved to have Maggie back. It was the first time we'd been apart since she was born. She ran through the living room into the kitchen, knelt, and gave me a big hug. "Teeny, school is so much fun! I'm gonna make sure Momma takes you tomorrow!"

"You all get in my room an' do y'r homework while I start dinner! No lazy dummies in my house!" yelled Momma, as she knelt and hugged me, too.

Momma took off her coat, and it covered the entire kitchen chair. "How was y'r day, Teeny?" she asked.

I looked at Daddy. Daddy looked at me. I understood right away that his age didn't mean a thing to Momma. She'd bust his head for fighting that cop.

"Well, Daddy went an' burnt th' eggs, but aside from that, it was all right, Momma," I responded cheerfully.

As Momma washed the dishes Daddy left in the sink, she huffed, "Humph! He burnt th' oatmeal, too!"

I twisted on that floor, desperately wanting to ask her, but decided to let her start the subject. She scrubbed that burnt pot and said, "Teeny, I talked to one of the counselors in school today and she told me that they have a new hospital that was built on the Boulevard for people like you. They even got a school there."

"Momma, can Maggie come with me?"

"No child, the school is just for you."

The day had been too much for me. I sobbed, "Well then, if she can't stay with me, who will take care of Maggie?"

WHO WILL TAKE CARE OF MAGGIE?

I watched Maggie and my cousins race out to school the next morning, then asked, "Momma, when will I get into that school on the Boulevard?"

"The counselor said it'll take about two weeks, if you want t' go, Teeny."

"Momma, I gotta think now, 'cause I can't leave Maggie."

Momma quickly washed me down with a rag and said, "I'm gonna take you next door to Miss Hippo's 'til I get back from th' farm. Your Daddy can't be with you today. He had to go to work. Now you stop worryin' so much about Maggie. Your not her mother, an' there's not too much you can do fa her."

"But I love her an' she loves me like I'm her mother. She even told me one day."

Momma just sighed. Then she picked me up in her big, strong arms and carried me to Miss Hippo's apartment. She laid me on a couch there and said, "You be good now. I'll be back in a few hours."

Miss Hippo asked Momma, "Does she need anything special to eat or anything?"

"She's able t' tell you how she goes to the bathroom an' anything else, Miss Hippo," Momma answered with a smile. Then she bent down, gave me a parting kiss, and left.

Miss Hippo sat next to me. She was so skinny. Why was she referred to as "Hippo"? Without a word, she reached over, grabbed a huge box of chocolates, and began to chomp. I watched. Eventually she asked, "Oh, want one, dearie?"

"Er—no thanks." I really loved chocolate, but the way she slobbered all over that candy, even the ones in the box, took away my appetite. Did she eat like that all the time?

Then, Miss Hippo did something that frightened me so that I would have raced away if I could. She took off her hair! All of it! Only a few red, bead–shaped curls were stuck to her snow–white scalp. I'd never seen anyone with such light skin, but such a flat nose and heavy lips. Years later I realized that this compulsive eater was an albino.

But right then, she drooled and chomped contentedly, then said, "I've heard a lot of nice things about you, Teeny."

"Yeah, what?"

She paused, "Er, y'r Daddy talks about you all the time. He's a real good, good, good man that daddy of yours. He truly is."

"Have you been knowing my Daddy for a long time? You got kids of y'r own?"

She was silent. She even stopped chomping on those chocolates. I watched; she sighed and bit her lip. "Yeah, Teeny, I got five."

Then she burst into tears. "I—I had to give 'em up for adoption!" She rubbed her chocolate–smeared fingers into her eyes. The couch shook with her sobbing.

Remembering the conversation two nights ago in Momma's kitchen, I asked fearfully, "Uh, why, Miss Hippo?"

"Cause the public assistance people kept sayin' they'd have a better chance than with me and no man."

"Where'd your husband go?"

"He's gone child, gone...."

"But where?" I persisted.

"He got up early every morning and tramped the streets, lookin' fa work. He was an A–one mechanic and even a chef. He spent five years lookin' fa work after he got busted for bein' near a robbed store. He didn't do it; I'd a'known if he had. Nobody would hire him. He sure loved his kids...."

"So where'd he go, Miss Hippo?"

"He jumped off the God–damned roof an' they took my kids!"

Something told me to shut up, but I just couldn't. "Er, but at least you get to see 'em...."

"No, the workers kept after me to sign 'em over for adoption, then when I did, they told me it was illegal fa me to see 'em anymore."

"Well, they got nice homes anyway, Miss Hippo."

"No, Betty Mae saw my Jim on the bus an' he said they was all split up in different foster homes. She said he looked awful shabby an' ashamed. But he jumped off the bus 'fore she could find out where he lived."

This time, instead of crying, she reached into the box and stuffed three chocolates into her mouth.

My mind reeled. Would the Welfare people take Maggie and put her in some shabby foster home? How come the workers kept after Miss Hippo to sign away her kids and then not let 'em be adopted? It was way over my head.

I watched and watched Miss Hippo stuff her face. Strange to say, she didn't offer to feed me any lunch, so I ate nothing. But I did get to see Captain Kangaroo, though he wasn't much fun without Maggie giggling next to me.

At last Daddy came in. Since the couch was facing the TV, he couldn't see me. He put his arms around Miss Hippo and said, "Let's not have any talk. Let's just go to bed."

She shoved him away with, "Watch y'r self. Don't you see y'r kid over there?"

Daddy groaned, "Oh Lord, I thought Momma had stayed home from work with her!"

Then he came over, picked me up, and gave me a kiss.

"Daddy, how come you got to go to bed now? It's time for us t' go now. G'bye Miss Hippo, an' thanks. See you later...I mean later...."

Back at Momma's, I just lay on my blanket in the kitchen watching Daddy as he began dinner. As usual he was humming, but this time, I didn't smell anything burning. I couldn't help laughing to myself, *Daddy's not like "Bachelor Father," because "Bachelor Father" never does any cooking.*

Soon we were invaded by Rose, Lloyd, Hank, Rusty, Adrian, Freddy, Bertha Mae, and Maggie. My cousins smiled and waved "Hi, Teeny!" then raced into the living room to their afternoon TV cartoons.

Maggie plopped down on the floor and held me around my neck. "I'm kinda mad, Teeny. Momma wouldn't take you to school with me today; after I'd promised you we'd go together." She pouted, "So I'm not ever goin back t'school again—unless Momma brings you, too."

I asked softly, "Didn't you have fun in school today, Maggie?"

"Yeah, it was all right, but all everybody did was play and do what the teacher said. School wasn't a lot of fun because nobody talked."

"Oh, makin' a good impression, growin' up, becoming a lady; you know, important things.

"You got to learn, Maggie, not everybody got the same things on their mind. And so some people like cartoons an' some people like old movies, like we do. But since we're not by ourselves anymore, we got to learn about other people."

"You can teach me, Teeny. Why do I haveta bother with those babies always jumpin' around?"

"Our not being together anymore hurts me. I'm not the only person in this world, Maggie. Just like on "'Gidget Grows Up'" she had to make it with new people too, remember?"

"She's all grown up already, Teeny!"

"Right, Maggie. But first, she had to go to school. And so, if you're sad an' all that, how you gonna help me with new people?"

"Why can't you come and learn with me?"

"Maggie, remember how everybody in the back of the bus, laughed at me? Well, the kids in any school are gonna laugh even more at me when the teacher has to stop everything just to take me to the bathroom Maggie, just think how awful that will be for me. Go to school for me, Maggie!"

"But Teeny if they laugh at you, I'll kick their butt!"

"Stop actin' like Mom now, like you can fight the whole school!"

Momma was standing in the kitchen doorway. "I hope you get the idea. You got to go to school without y'r sister. She'll go to a special place an' learn to read also. You two can't be Siamese twins all your lives. God won't allow it."

My cousins filed in for dinner. Maggie handed me my plate. Then she watched me eat with my mouth as she always did. Then she watched our cousins as they sat and ate with amazement. She ate practically nothing.

Even Momma retired early, and I was alone with the sound of her snoring.

"Momma! Let me in!" came from the hallway. The front door shook as someone banged on it. "Momma! Momma!"

Momma woke up and stared. "What in the world's happenin'?"

"Somebody's at the door callin' you, Momma!" I said.

The racket continued. She trudged to the door and opened it.

"Where you been all this time, Anita?"

I crawled to the edge of the bed and watched. So that's my Aunt Anita! My grandmother picked up Hank's halfball stick and charged toward a dark woman whose enormous breasts were half covered by a flimsy frilled blouse. She repeated, "Where the hell you been? How could you leave your own kids for so damn long?"

My aunt backed away from the door and yelled, "Momma, I'm not gonna let you hit me with that stick!"

"Hit you? I should kill you!" She yelled again, "Anita, Anita! Where have you been? Where have you been?"

That big–busted woman smirked, "I've been at a card game."

"For three days? Are you crazy?"

"Well, Momma, you just gotta learn how I take care of business." With that, Anita opened her huge shopping bag and dumped piles, and piles, and piles of money on the kitchen table. It just seemed like the stack of money got higher each time another pile of money was added to it.

Momma whooped, "How the hell you get all this money?" She scooped up a fist–full of bills. "Why, there aren't all ones here. You got tens an' twenties an' even a fifty dollar bill here!"

Very nonchalantly, Anita said, "Sure, they'se over two–thousand bucks here. It takes time to make money like that, Momma."

"You been out shopliftin' again, huh?"

"No, I had enough of that, Momma. I got no intention of goin' t' jail again. It's like I said; gamblin'—an' a couple other things have led to this pile of money that I wish would go on and on forever."

Momma put down the stick and sat down. "None of my kids gonna join me in heaven!"

"Momma, I am not about t' be insulted by no bitch who works for welfare no more."

"Don't use that kinda talk in my house," Momma ordered as she sorted the bills into neat piles.

"Hey, Anita's here!" cried Rose coming into the kitchen.

They stumbled into the kitchen, rubbing the sleep from their eyes and squinting at the light. First they stared, without approaching their mother. Then Rose, the eldest, moaned, "Where have you been gone to for so long, Anita?"

"I been findin' ways t' keep you kids from starvin', see!" she pointed to the money on the table, then held out her arms. "Now come an' kiss me."

Her children looked at all that money and rushed to her, kissing and hugging. An outsider would have thought she'd just come home from work a few hours late. The kitchen was filled with shouts of "Anita's back! Anita's back!" Maggie stumbled in, half asleep.

"What's she doin' here, Momma? Where's Frances?" Anita asked.

Momma answered, "We don't know where she is. Their Daddy picked 'em up from the jailhouse. The cops was chasin' Frances an' that woman–friend of hers, but we don't know what for."

Anita sneered, "Oh, Frances on the run again, that fool! She's just not slick enough yet."

My sister winced. Our cousins watched.

Anita continued, "You all get back t' bed. I'm takin' you home tomorrow."

My cousins clapped, "We gonna go home! Good night, Anita."

"Goodnight!" she replied, and they skipped back to bed.

My sister trudged behind them, without a word.

Anita sighed, "Whew, I'm tired! I'll just bunk with you, Momma."

Before Momma could answer, my aunt had switched on the bedroom light and yelled, "Oh, what do we do about her?"

I said, "Goodnight, Anita."

I heard a rude, "Hello, Teeny," before she swung back to the kitchen. "You know Momma, that kid was wide awake, listenin' an lookin' at everything from the end of the bed."

"She never seems t' sleep very much. But she got a lot t' worry about, where her mother is; how the hell she herself gonna survive, an' who's gonna take care of Maggie when they'se separated."

"Well, they ain't my kids. I'm tired. I'm gonna sleep in that bed, too. How you gonna squeeze into that small bed, Momma?"

"I'm not. I got to go to the farm in an hour, anyway. So I'll just put my feet up here an' try to rest."

"You don't haveta go to no farm, Momma. You see I got. money."

"Yeah, I see it. I'll take what you give me for those three days with your kids. But there's no guarantee that you'll be able t' give out money like that all the time. So I better keep my job. It's regular, honest pay, an' I'm not beholdin' to a soul."

"If you want t' be that way about it, good night!" Anita came in, snatched off her skirt and that frilly blouse. I peeked at those huge breasts. But I was too tired to contemplate whether I'd ever look like that and soon fell asleep.

Voices in the kitchen awakened me. "No school this morning. Just get yer things together 'cause we goin' home when Momma gets back frum work."

"Howcum there's no school?" Maggie asked.

"Don't you see the snow piled high? On the radio they called y'r school closed today."

"Oh, okay. Let me go see if Teeny wants her cereal," Maggie said then came into the bedroom smiling. "Sugar Pops or plain Corn Flakes, Teeny?" Then she giggled, "I hid the pops so they wouldn't eat 'em all up."

"Gee thanks, Maggie." Soon I was chomping on that rare treat, with all that sugar I didn't need but which tasted so great.

Maggie left me to help with the dishes. I watched as she and my cousins fought over whose turn it was, then to dry. I remembered those few happy times with my own mother when she would lay me on the kitchen floor, put one dishtowel in back of me, and another one in my feet. Then she would place a few dishes in back of me and say, "Dry 'em, Teeny."

I'd rub one side of each dish, turn it over with my toes, dry the other side, and lift it to the dry pile. Would anyone ever grant me' "my turn" at doing dishes again?

Soon Anita opened the front door, for the mailman had slipped letters under it. She picked up the mail and said, "Oh! Hi, Mr. Cain. How's Agnes an' the kids?"

A bass–voiced, unfriendly man answered, "They'se fine," and a huge, dark–skinned man in a greasy garage outfit stepped inside. It was my mother's father, whom we called "Daddy Cain."

"What brings you to our part of the world?" Anita ventured.

Maggie ran over, "Daddy Cain, we ain't seen you in so long. You still got that big car?"

Daddy Cain picked her up and hugged her slightly. He wasn't much for kissing. Then, "Where's Teeny at?" he asked.

Maggie pointed to the bedroom.

He put her down and entered. I said, "Hi, Daddy Cain. Did Mom tell you where she's at?"

"No, she just wants you with us," he answered shortly.

"When she comin' back?"

"Look, Teeny, don't bother me with no questions. I got enough t' figure out."

Anita entered.

"Mister Cain, you can't take these kids 'til Momma comes home. I can't just let 'em go."

"Look girl, I took a whole day off a good construction job to come get 'em an' I'm takin' 'em now. Get you an' y'r sister's clothes together, Maggie."

Maggie ran out. My cousin, Rose, said to her, "Gee, it's kinda sad we got to be split up. We got to know each other pretty good, tho' it wasn't for long."

"Don't worry. Daddy Cain will bring us back to visit, won't you, Daddy Cain?" Maggie asked.

My grandfather muttered, "We'll see about that."

Soon, Maggie and I were bundled up and ready to go again. Daddy Cain picked me up and let all my cousins kiss and hug me, as well as Maggie.

"'Bye, Rose; 'Bye, Adrian; 'Bye, Hank; 'Bye, Rusty; 'Bye, Freddy; 'Bye, Bertha Mae; Bye, Lloyd. I promise I'll be back to visit!" Not being able to say goodbye to our father or our Momma, hurt badly. Would we ever enjoy such great cooking again?

Finally we tore ourselves from our cousins and left the apartment. "Oh, don't start down yet, Daddy Cain. I gotta say goodbye to Miss Hippo. She took care of me while Momma went to the farm."

"Okay," was the deep approval. Maggie knocked on Miss Hippo's door. It was open. The smell of whiskey came to us before Miss Hippo appeared with a huge box of chocolates in her hand. Jesus! All she had on was a pair of underpants. "Er, er, I'm leavin' now, Miss Hippo. G'bye," I managed to get out, despite the shock.

"What you tellin' me for? You ain't one of my kids," she sobbed. She swayed from side to side, then slammed the door. Daddy Cain took us down those three long flights of stairs. At the front door, Maggie said, "Gee, there's a big spot on that floor—looks like blood, Teeny."

I looked down and said, "You got some imagination, Maggie. Somebody probably spilled some ketchup."

We entered the winter atmosphere. It felt wonderful. I hadn't been out for days. Making rings of my warm breath into the cold air was pure joy. Maggie understood. She bent down, picked up some snow, made a snowball, and heaved it at my head. She missed. I wish she hadn't.

"Stop the foolishness," Daddy Cain ordered. He opened the rear of his station wagon and slid me inside. "Sit next to y'r sister an' make sure she doesn't fall."

"I know all about that, Daddy Cain. You don't have t' tell me," Maggie said as she hopped in beside me.

Soon we were in a neighborhood of tall, bare trees and proud, old homes with beautiful porches! There were areas where the homes were made of stone built to last forever.

"Where are we, Daddy Cain?" I asked.

"Germantown," was his answer.

Some streets were not paved but cobbled. Some homes had miles of forbidding steps before one dared reach their huge front doors. Others stood flush with the street, tiny and humble, revealing their age with their ancient shutters.

Daddy Cain angled that huge station wagon down an impossible narrow street that was once a steep hill. Each house clung to its neighbor, each roof pointed one step lower than the next, until the last roof appeared to touch the ground. But each home had its own porch, its special garden, its independent color determined by the personality of its owner.

In the middle of the street, kids yelled, "Whoops! Whee!" as they sled down into the city's snow.

I watched and thought, *I've been carried through the snow, but how does snow feel? It must be cold, but a friendly cold.*

Daddy Cain pulled to the curb. The car half–covered the middle of the street. He opened the back and Maggie jumped out. I tried to slip to the edge by myself, but heard a deep, "Watch it, Miss Freshy!" He lifted me out and picked his way through the piles of snow. I could feel the crunch of his heavy boots. We made our way up the high stairs of one of those tiny row houses. "Push the bell, Maggie. I can't reach m' keys holdin' her."

"Okay, Daddy Cain," she said and did so. Soon someone came to the door who looked exactly as my mother would in a decade or so. She grabbed Maggie, kissed her, then hugged the breath out of her. "Oh, God, you're safe!"

My mother's mother, who we also called "Mom," looked at me as Daddy Cain tramped in the house and set me, not too gently, on the couch. She sat on the floor beside me, then hugged and kissed me, too. "Oh, chile, are you cold?"

"No, Mom, I love the winter."

As she removed my coat, she fussed about my mother. "I don't know what's wrong with that daughter of mine. She was only fourteen when she went an' sold the lease to this house right from under us to white people. Just to get one hundred dollars fa clothes. It wasn't like she was naked, but she always had to have more. She's been that way ever since."

She looked at Maggie, then back at me. I bowed my head. She said softly, "Well, now I got a chance to do a little better."

I felt relieved. She wanted us.

Slam! "Mom, who's that Daddy Cain brought out of the car?"

"Mom, who we got here?"

"Mom, why she layin' on the couch, steada playin' in the snow?"

"Mom!" "Mom!" "Mom!" with many questions and curious looks came from about nine children, ranging in age from five to twelve.

I cringed. Oh, God, more kids to stare at me as I ate with my mouth.

"Stop yellin' an' meet y'r aunts, uncles, and cousins!' She pulled Maggie to her and said, "Maggie gonna be livin' here 'til your sister Frances come fa her. Teeny may be livin' in a school, unless she or Frances don't like it. But this is Teeny an' Maggie's regular home now. Get it?"

A huge ton dropped from my shoulders. I was certain that this mom would never let Maggie be shoved into any foster home. Maggie would always be safe.

Mom introduced us to her four children who had not as yet left home. Their friends looked on curiously. My little sister drew close to me defensively.

Mom's children were Bobby, age seventeen, the philosopher who worked after school; Libby, age eight, the household bookworm; Craig, age seven, the kleptomaniac; and Lenny, age five. He was the youngest, and therefore, the spoiled brat. The names of their friends floated over my head. I would sort them out later.

One of their friends asked, "Mom, Maggie an' Teeny come out in the snow now?" (All the neighbors' kids called my grandmother "Mom.")

Maggie said, "Teeny can't go in the snow."

Libby asked, "Why not?"

"Because she can't walk right now. But she'll walk when she's a lady."

Mom looked startled, but said nothing. Libby continued, "How old is she?"

"She's six, an' I'm five."

Lenny took his thumb out of his mouth to butt in. "She's older'n me an' I been walkin'."

Craig sneered, "Hmmm, she's just stupid, layin' there."

Mom yelled, "Stop it! She's not stupid. She just can't walk an' I don't want no more talk about it!"

I said, "That's all right, Mom, they'll learn."

Bobby, the eldest, said, "You see, she can talk."

Daddy Cain re—entered the room. "Maggie, when the snow clears tomorrow morning, I gonna take you to Henry School. You got enough papers 'n stuff?"

"Yes, Daddy Cain! Where is Teeny goin'?"

"When I talked with your other grandma, she said Teeny's goin' to the school on the Boulevard."

"Oh, yeah, but I kept hopin' things would change when we got here," Maggie explained sadly. "But Daddy Cain, can I go with you to Teeny's school first just to see it? I can start my school after that, please?"

Maggie and I looked all the way up to our gruff grandfather. He looked all the way down to us and said, "Guess so," then walked out.

Soon it was lunchtime. My grandmother had never been confronted with the idea of caring for me. So she laid me on a sheet on the kitchen table. "Here's y'r sandwich, chile. Now eat it all." She cut it into small pieces and proceeded to feed it to me, piece by piece.

"No, Mom, I'll do it myself. Just lay it in front of me."

Mom stopped feeding me. Then she and her children stared until I had picked up each piece with my mouth.

Lenny yelped, "She eats like a dog!"

Whack! Mom slapped him in the face. "Don't you dare make fun of her, no more, no time. She can't use her arms nor legs! I hope you all understand now."

There was no more conversation.

That night Maggie and I slept together again. Who would know that it would be for the last time in our childhoods? We were worried.

"How they gonna treat you in that special school, Teeny?"

"Who gonna tell you when to be quiet, Maggie?"

"Are lotsa people gonna hurt y'r feelings there, Teeny?"

"Who gonna explain the TV shows to you when you fall asleep after commercials, Maggie?"

And worst of all, "Where's our own mom? Daddy Cain wouldn't say a word about her."

The next morning I lay on the kitchen table and watched my young aunts and uncles prepare for school. Maggie gathered up her brand–new note pads and well–pointed pencils and placed them in a pretty plastic container Mom had found "from her kids now gone." (Mom had only five of her original thirteen children alive. Some of the others had died along the way, most of them tragically.)

Maggie said, "Grandpa's gonna take us to the Boulevard School soon. He says that if you like it, he's gonna leave you there. I hope you don't like it, then you can stay with me."

"Isn't that kinda selfish? I gotta learn too, Maggie."

"Yeah, you're right, Teeny. At least I'll get to visit you."

Soon we were in the station wagon. The snow was almost gone, and the streets were filled with ice. But when we got on the Benjamin Franklin Parkway, each car zoomed past as though it was bent on self–destruction. We were terrified. Maggie cried.

"We here," Daddy Cain muttered. He lifted me out. As we came up the walk of the special hospital, the doors swung open automatically.

Maggie laughed, in spite of her sorrow. "Somebody must be watchin' out 'specially fa you, Teeny!"

Daddy Cain carried me into the office and announced, "I got Celestine Tate."

A dumpy woman with all–white face powder and steel–dyed hair responded, "Well, here is our new student."

5 THE MEDICAL MAZE

"Doctor Sawyer, Doctor Sawyer," I heard over the loud intercom.

The receptionist said to my grandfather, "Come this way, Mr. Tate."

He said, "Cain is my name; this is my granddaughter."

My grandfather carried me into a big office. As I was looking over my grandfather's shoulders, still seeing my sister holding the back of his coat, the receptionist said, "Have a seat."

Before sitting down, my grandfather put me on the floor as he always did.

The receptionist asked my grandfather, "Does she sit in a wheel-chair?"

Being use to my grandfather and not saying much, he just said, "No, her back don't bend."

She said, "Wait just a minute, I'll see if I can find her a litter."

Always remembering what I learned on TV, I thought she was going to put me in a trash can.

She came back wheeling a bed with four wheels. The receptionist said, "Lay her on here, Mr. Cain."

My grandfather laid me on the litter on my stomach.

Looking back at my sister, wondering why she was so quiet, watching her pull her buttons off her coat as she always did, my grandfather looked over at her and said, "Get over here, girl; ain't you learned how to unbutton your coat yet? Now go over there and help your sister take off her coat."

Maggie always had a harder time taking off my clothes than her own, but with both of us working together, she eventually got them off.

The receptionist said, "I have a few questions to ask you, Mr. Cain." She reached in her big desk, which looked like a dining room table to me, and pulled out a folder. She asked him for my birthdate.

After hearing him say, Uh..., uh..., uh ...," I knew he didn't know. "October 15th," I shouted.

"What hospital was she born in?" was her next question.

When I found myself answering the second question by myself, I felt smarter than my own grandfather.

She finally asked me a question I couldn't answer. "Have you been immunized?"

I told her, "I don't know what you mean."

"Have you had your shots?" she replied.

I told her the only shots I had were the shots they give us when the big blue truck comes around the neighborhood.

The receptionist said to my grandfather, "Sign this form Mr. Cain, we can get the rest of the information from her medical records."

I watched as my grandfather reached in his shirt pocket and took out his bifocals that he got from a five and ten; he never spent more than 20 or 30 cents for his glasses. At that moment, a white man with a long white coat came into the office.

"Oh, there you are, Dr. Sawyers," the receptionist shouted.

"Here is our new student, Celestine Tate," she said.

My grandfather quickly stood up and took his dirty baseball cap off his head and shook the doctor's hand.

"Cain is my name," he said, "and I'm glad to know she can go to school. Do ya'll give 'em three meals a day here?" was his next question.

Even as miserly as my grandfather was, he always made sure we had something to eat.

"They sure do, Mr. Cain; we take good care of them here." The doctor grabbed the bed I was laying on and started to pull it.

My grandfather laid our coats on the stretcher then grabbed the other end.

I said, "Daddy Cain, don't forget about Maggie."

"Come on, girl, you see us leaving," he said.

Maggie then ran over to my grandfather and grabbed his long, dirty, grey coat, rubbing her eyes with her left hand. Before long we were up the hallway into the classroom.

There were a whole mess of wheelchairs and beds in there. All the children looked strange to me, nothing like I was used to, but it really didn't matter. Finally being in my own classroom was the only thing I really looked forward to.

Then another white lady came up to me and said, "Who do we have here?"

The doctor said, "This is our new student; her name is Celestine Tate."

The lady replied, "How old are you, Celestine?"

"Six years old," I answered.

She said happily, "Good, you'll be in my class. My name is Mrs. Desedaris, but all the kids call me Mrs. D.O."

She was exceptionally tall to be a lady, with red hair and tiny wire—framed glasses.

My teacher then said, "Excuse me, Timmy wants me."

With my eyes on all the kids, not seeing one or more raise their hands or hearing someone speaking, I wondered how she knew that Timmy wanted her.

She went over to a little white boy who was sitting in a wheelchair shaking his leg vigorously, gathering in my mind that shaking his leg in that way was his way of raising his hand.

I was very excited; it looked like a real classroom to me. It had blackboards and everything.

Doctor Sawyer said, "Wait right here, Mr. Cain." Then he trotted up the hall and shut off the crying by closing the door.

Then he came back to me, and I asked him, "Who was crying and why?"

"It's just a little boy who wants his mommy, he'll be all right. The nurse is in there with him. Here is the gym."

They rolled me into another big room. I liked this room, too. It had lots of toys, weights, wooden stair steps, and mats all over the floor. I was liking the school even more knowing that I could sit on the floor sometimes, although I was kind of worried about that because of the way the receptionist looked at my grandfather for laying me on the floor.

The doctor said, "You can come here everyday and get your exercise."

Doctor Sawyer said to my grandfather, "Come this way, Mr. Cain; I have to talk to you for a minute."

My grandfather then bent down and picked up Maggie and sat her on the bed where I was laying and said, "Wait here with Teeny; I'll be right back."

Maggie then said, "Teeny, do you like it here? Are you staying?"

"Yes, I'm going to stay Maggie, because I'm going to learn so that I can teach you. Anyway they'll let me out Fridays and Saturdays, and I'll come and visit you every week, plus you know what we agreed on, always to be together at Christmas. And I know you saw Mom putting up the Christmas tree when we left. Christmas is on Sunday you know, we'll be together soon! You just wait and see."

My grandfather came back in and said, "Teeny, are you going to be alright here?"

I said, "Yes, Daddy Cain. I think I'm going to make it here."

Maggie jumped down off the bed where I was laying, ran out of the room straight down the hall, and out the double doors.

My grandfather said to the doctor, "Don't mind her; I don't know what's wrong with her. Let me get her coat. I know it's cold out there."

He yelled back to me, "I'll come see you as soon as they say I can,

Teeny."

Grandfather quickly shook the doctor's hand and said, "Thank you for all your trouble." Then he raced out to get Maggie.

Doctor Sawyer said, "I'm going to take you to your bedroom now." He wheeled me into a room with beds going all the way up one side and down the other. He pushed me up next to a bed that had bars all around it like a crib.

I asked him, "Why did I have to have a bed with bars around it. I'm not going to fall?"

He then said, "It's a safety precaution; it's the rules."

Doctor Sawyer then asked me, "How do I pick you up?"

I answered, "Just put the stretcher near the bed; I can get on it myself." I then asked him if I would be able to go to school now.

He quickly responded, "No, the nurse will be in, in a minute."

After the doctor helped me into the bed, and put up the side rail on it, I laid and thought, *Why does this school have nurses and doctors? I bet this place is a hospital, and they are probably cutting that little boy over there wide open, and that's why he is crying.*

At that moment a nurse came in my room I and asked me if I had my lunch.

I said, "Yes, I had greens, potato salad, and chicken."

She said, "Oh, you won't be eating those types of foods here."

She then told me, "Turn over if you can; I have to take your clothes off. The doctors want to examine you."

"Why do doctors want to see me? I came here to go to school."

The nurse replied, "Don't argue. Those are the rules." She rudely said, "Who brought you in?"

I told her my grandfather did, and she said, "It doesn't matter—he's gone. Your chart will be up in a few minutes. I can get your address and send him your clothes."

"Why are you going to send him my clothes. I need my clothes?"

"You have to wear the hospital's clothes. Don't argue!"
Those are the rules.

I said to myself, *I knew it was a hospital all of the time.*

As she was struggling to get my arms into the hospital gown, a whole lot of doctors in white coats came in. I had been stripped bare, feeling very strange around all these men with nothing on but a nightgown. I saw Doctor Sawyer and then he came up to me and said to all the doctors, "This is Celestine Tate, our new patient. I haven't examined her yet." Then he pulled up my hand that was folded across my chest. "Seeing her webbed fingers indicates to me the fact that she has a congenital disease now and should be under experimental means of a cure. The medical term is called Arthrogryposis Multiplex. She is one of our first cases. I hope your interns learn a lot from her. She's also exceptionally bright," he said as he rubbed his head. All the other doctors turned and walked out mumbling to each other.

Doctor Sawyer said, "I'll be seeing you in a little while; you rest now."

As soon as he walked away, I quickly turned back on my stomach. Watching him and his doctor friends through the nurse's window writing in something, I knew right away it was a chart. I watched a lot of "General Hospital."

The nurse came back in the room and said to me, "They're not going to do anything else to you, so you can go to school this afternoon."

To me that was the best thing she could have said.

I said, "What about my clothes?"

She rapidly spoke out and said, "We don't have time for that; I'll just put a sheet over you."

I was on my back in Mrs. D.O.'s class. A man in a blue suit had taken me there.

Mrs. D.O. said, "I'm glad you came back. I wanted to introduce you to the class." She went behind her desk and tapped her pencil three times, and said, "Class, I'd like for you to meet Celestine Tate. She is our new student."

Everybody all at once yelled, jumped, and wiggled their words of hello to me. Then Mrs. D.O. came over and gave me a board with a paper on it. She asked me could I write.

I softly whispered, "A little bit; you just have to put a pencil in my mouth."

She did as I suggested and then asked me if I knew how to count.

My answer was, "A little bit."

She said, "Count the apples and put the answer in the box."

Mrs. D.O. inquired, "Can you write your name?"

I said, "Yes!"

My teacher then directed me to write my name on every paper I received up on the line.

She politely said, "If you write your name, and it is correct, you'll get a gold star. That's an 'A' in my class."

And then I got very excited about getting a gold star. I was determined to get a gold star on every paper. Then I bent down to write my name and put in the answer. The paper just wouldn't hold still. I raised my pencil, and Mrs. D.O. came over to me. I told her the paper just wouldn't hold still.

"Here, I'll put it in the clip of the board."

I held the paper still, but yet my writing still looked awfully crooked.

Mrs. Desedaris decided that my pencil must be too long. She broke it in half and we sharpened it, then erased what I had done.

She said, "Try again; I think you'll do better now."

Sharpening the pencil did the trick, now I was on my way. I was rushing to get finished so I could get my gold star.

Then the school bell rang, and Mrs. D.O. said to the class, "Don't forget to do your homework."

I said, "I'm not finished yet."

She responded, "Take it to your room and finish it."

I knew if I had until tomorrow, I was sure to get a gold star.

Five or six white men came into the classroom and started pulling out the wheelchairs and beds. One of the men in blue grabbed my bed and started to pull.

My teacher said, "Leave her here; I have to test her."

Soon the class was empty. Mrs. D.O. came over to me and said, "Let me see what you've done so far? You have everything right so far." Then she asked me, "Who taught you how to count?"

I told her my mother's boyfriend, Sandy, taught me how to count those funny little cigarettes that my mother rolled all by herself.

Then my teacher asked me if I knew my A–B–C's. I told her I didn't think so. I recited them for her as much as I remembered from being taught on "Romper Room."

She said, "Here, take this paper, put your name on it, and fill in the missing letters. And I'll see you tomorrow in hopes of giving you that gold star."

Soon I was back in the ward, only now the ward was full of children. There was a white girl in the bed next to me with short blonde hair who had no arms or legs.

She said, "You just came in today?"

I said, "Yes!" I asked her, "Is this a hospital?"

She said, "It sure is; they fooled me, too."

She asked me what my name was, and I told her. "But my friends call me, Teeny."

She said, "My name is Pat."

Then I asked her how old she was, and she told me she was eight years old.

I asked her if they cut people open in here.

She shouted, "They sure do."

The nurse came in and clapped her hands three times, then she said, "Everybody get to their beds; the dinner truck is coming."

That was something I understood; I was very hungry.

Finally a big steel truck came up the elevator with stacks of trays on it. The nurse and an assistant pulled the truck into the middle of the ward.

The nurse yelled, "Spaghetti tonight!"

I love spaghetti, I thought to myself.

She reached into the side of the truck and picked up a huge spoon and started dipping out the spaghetti onto the tray. Her assistant would carry the tray to the patient's beds.

Everybody was soon eating. She pulled the truck out of the room and she came back with a silver sign and hung it on my bed.

I asked her, "Why don't I get anything to eat?"

She informed me, "You have to get your blood taken in the morning."

I yelled, "But I'm hungry!"

She then nodded saying, "Those are the rules; don't argue!"

I turned over on my back and started crying to myself. I never could cry out loud for fear Maggie would hear me. I remembered what my Grandma Cain said to me; "Always think of something happy when you're sad." So I did.

I was back at my mother's house on Christmas day. Maggie had woken me up. She said, "It's Christmas, come on, let's go see what we got."

She took the cover off me, then she picked me up putting her left hand under my neck and her right hand through my folded legs, and struggled to carry me to the living room. She turned on the light and there was the tree with nothing under it. Now I was just as disappointed as Maggie.

Maggie ran into my mother's room and I heard her little voice say, "Where's Santa Claus? Didn't he come?"

Mom said, "It's too early for Santa Claus, so back to bed. Where's Teeny?"

Maggie told her, "She's in the living room."

My mother asked, "How did Celestine get there?"

Maggie said, "I carried her."

Mother said, "Well, you just get your behind in there carry her back."

Maggie came back into the room to carry me to bed, then we heard a knock at the door. Mother answered it.

"Ho, Ho, Ho," I heard. "Merry Christmas."

Maggie ran over and sat down beside me and she said, "Teeny, it's Santa Claus."

And sure enough it was. He came in with a big red bag. I knew it was full of toys. He came in and sat down and he picked me up and sat down, and laid me across his lap. Then he asked me what I wanted for Christmas.

I told him, "I want a doll, games, and a stove." Every toy I named he pulled out of the bag. There was something funny about this Santa Claus. He had the white beard and the big stomach and all, but I felt as though I knew him from somewhere.

He then put me down and picked up Maggie. He asked Maggie if she had been a good girl.

She said, "Yes," and gave him a great big hug. Maggie then put her hand over her mouth and started giggling, pulled Santa Claus's beard, I and said, "Teeny, it's only Daddy," and we laughed and laughed.

"Study hour," I heard the nurse shout. Now I was out of my dream and back at the hospital. I felt kind of happy again. The last Christmas was the best Christmas I ever had. Now I could study and get my gold star for tomorrow.

"Eight o'clock, time to get ready for bed," the nurse said.

They undressed all the children and put them into bed. I remember missing Maggie very much, and crying myself to sleep.

I was awakened by a fat nurse. She put the side rail down on my bed and said, "C'mon. Hop on the stretcher. I have to take you downstairs to see the doctor."

I looked around the ward and saw that all the kids were gone. I asked the nurse where they had gone. She said they had gone to class. I was very disappointed because I wanted to get my gold star.

She rolled me down the hall and onto the elevator and went downstairs. It was a whole different sight. There were a lot of machines and everything was green. She took me into a big room where there were about ten doctors.

Dr. Sawyer said, "Here's our star patient, Celestine Tate. She has Arthrogryposis Multiplex, a congenital disease that affects the nervous system of the body. Notice her webbed fingers."

I was laying there listening to these big words, wondering what it all meant.

My doctor said, "Well, what are you planning to do with her?"

Doctor Sawyer said, "Her case is very rare. There hasn't been anything done yet, but God, we're going to try."

"From what I hear, she's extremely intelligent. If we can't do anything for her body, we're sure going to do something for her mind."

They continued to talk about medical things that I didn't understand.

The nurse came back and announced, "We're ready to take the test now."

The doctors followed as she pushed me out of the room into another room.

Suddenly I saw another nurse coming towards me. She had a blood pressure kit and wrapped it around my arm real tight. I was wondering what was going on. She brought out a big needle and I became very frightened. I started to cry.

Dr. Sawyer said, "It doesn't hurt a bit." He took the needle and said, "Well, I'll do it."

It reminded me of the time my Uncle Clement stabbed my Uncle Bobby in the stomach. I felt as though I was being stabbed, too.

After that they laid me on a big round table. A man in a green suit walked in. He stood in front of an old–fashioned camera shaped like a box with three legs holding it up. He put a slide into the camera and turned the machine on.

The table on which I was lying turned around very slowly. He picked up a cord from the floor and squeezed something on it and the camera clicked. He took that slide out and put more in. The camera kept clicking and my table kept moving. I felt like I was on a merry–go–round. I enjoyed it.

The doctors were still mumbling and talking. They stopped the table and picked me up and put me on my knees and leaned me against the wall. The camera started clicking again and more pictures were taken. Then they turned me around so that my face was against the wall. They took more pictures, and I didn't have on any clothes, just a diaper strung up around my waist. I was so frightened.

Doctor Sawyer picked me up and put me back on the stretcher. I was put into another room. He said, "This test is going to be a little painful, but it won't hurt that much." They took out a metal–ring that looked like a hat and put it on my head. Then they attached a lot of wire strips with sticky stuff on the ends to the bar that was around my head.

Dr. Sawyer took the needles that were in the wires and stuck them into my head under the first layer of skin, and I screamed.

Doctor Sawyer said, "We're going to give you a brain scan."

They turned on a machine that had a wave going across it. The machine was ticking away; I saw the needle jump higher as I got nervous. He tore off the strip of paper that had my brain waves on it. He said that it was to be taken down to the lab and read right away.

Then he began to remove the needles and other contraptions off of my head. I started to feel very weak and hungry, and I wanted to go home.

As I was lying in the room waiting for the doctors to come back there, I thought about how the other kids must be having fun in school and how I wished I was there instead of here. I thought to myself, *Why did they bring me to a hospital? I just want to go to school. I didn't come here for all this. Just wait 'til Maggie finds out.*

They came back and said, "You can go back to your room now."

By the time I got back to my room, it was lunchtime. All the children were coming back. They were bringing back the wheelchairs and stretchers. Everybody looked very cheerful and happy. I didn't feel very well at all. I had a headache, I felt dizzy, and I was hungry. The food cart came in, and I was wondering if they were going to feed me or starve me to death.

The lady said, "Ravioli, today?"

Ravioli! I'd never heard of that before. *I hope it's good and I hope I get some*, I thought.

The nurse came up to me and said, "Tate, are you ready to eat?"

I quickly said, "Yes!"

She put my food down in front of me.

She said, "They sent up a special cup for you today because the other cups are too heavy for you."

She gave me a cup that looked like a toy coffee pot. I sucked out of the spout and the milk came out. I ate ravioli for the first time, and it was good. I asked the nurse if I would be able to go back to class with the rest of the kids.

She said, "Yes, but since they don't have the time to dress you, you have to go in your gown."

I didn't mind. I was just glad to go.

Soon we were all off to school again. I was looking forward to seeing Mrs. D.O. again because I had finished my work and knew it was all right.

When we got to class Mrs. D.O. said, "Glad to see you back, Celestine."

"I'm very anxious for you to see my homework."

She said, "Just a minute."

I quickly looked over my work to see that everything was all right. I wasn't sure if the "p" was in the right place, or if the "q" was in the right place.

The teacher looked my work over and gave me another slip and told me what to do.

There was a little boy in the room. He had wet himself, and all the children were laughing.

Mrs. D.O. looked rather upset. She clapped her hands and told them to be quiet.

I thought to myself, *He is kind of big to be wetting his pants.* But for some reason, I didn't find it funny. She said that he could not help what he was doing. Mrs. D.O. pushed him out of the classroom, and one of the men came to take him to his room.

The janitor came and cleaned up the mess.

Mrs. D.O. started writing on the board.

She said, "Does anybody know what 1 and 1 is ?"

I quickly shouted, "Two."

"Very good."

Then she went on to repeat the numbers, two plus two, three plus three, and so on. It started to get difficult, so I quieted down. Most of the kids in my class seemed very smart. Mrs. D.O. came over to me and gave me back my piece of paper. I turned it over and saw I had two wrong, but she still gave me a gold star.

I told myself that every paper I turned into her would get a gold star. The bell rang. All the kids put their hands up and said goodbye to Mrs. D.O.

I said, "Will I get a gold star?"

She said, "If you get it all right."

Everybody went back to their room.

The nurse said, "Study hour" as soon as we got back to the room, so I had time to finish what I had started in class. She came up to me and put a sign on my bed. I couldn't see it.

My girlfriend, Peggy, said, "It says NOTHING BY MOUTH."

I said, "Oh, no, not again! You mean I can't eat breakfast?"

Peggy asked me what they had done to me today and I told her.

"That means they are going to operate on you tomorrow, she said.

"Operate?" I started screaming hysterically.

The nurse came running in, asking what was wrong?

"Peggy says the doctor is going to operate on me tomorrow. Is that true? Is that true?"

The nurse said, "Yes, the doctors are going to fix your arm."

I told her, "I don't want my arm fixed. I just want to go to school."

She said, "Well, your mother was here today, and she signed for you to get this operation.

I was so upset because my mother had come to the hospital and didn't even stay to see me. Plus thinking the whole night through that I was going to get an operation even though I didn't want to didn't make me the least bit happy. And I thought to myself that when I was old enough I could say no and then they couldn't do it to me ever again.

Early the next morning, before the children awakened, they came and got me, put me on a stretcher, and rolled me down the hall. Before I knew it, they gave me two needles. I started to feel dizzy and sleepy. They rolled me into a room and put me on a hard table. There were doctors and nurses standing all around, dressed in green. The nurse picked up a mask and put it over my face. I felt like I was being smothered to death and there was nothing I could do. I felt like I was dying and would never see Maggie again. How sad to think that I might die and nobody, I mean no family members, were even by my side. What a sad feeling to know that you are all alone, but even in this lonely time, I knew inside of myself that God was still with me.

When she removed the mask from my face, I was asleep; but I was not asleep because I could hear everything that the doctor was saying yet I couldn't feel what they were doing. I was thinking in my mind about whether or not I could open my eyes if I wanted to. I tried, but I couldn't. I felt them pulling on my arm, but I didn't feel any pain. My whole body was numb. I couldn't even wiggle my toes.

Suddenly I found the strength to open my eyes. I saw a lot of blood gushing out of my arm. Both of my arms were up in my face, and now my arm was down on my stomach. I thought to myself, *How do they know I want my arm there? I liked it where it was.*

The nurse looked at me and said, "Oh, she's awake. She has to be put back to sleep."

They put the mask back over my face. When I awoke again I was in another room with my arm all wrapped up. I remember feeling thirsty. They told me that I couldn't have any water. The nurse wet a rag, and I sucked the rag.

After a few days they asked me how I felt. They told me I was able to go back to my room. I wanted to go back with the other kids, but the doctor told me he didn't think I was ready. I insisted that I was, so he took me to my room and I felt very sick and nauseated. The loud noise of the kids talking and playing really upset me.

So they took me back to the recovery room that night. The doctors said that they couldn't do much more for me because I couldn't take it.

I don't know why my mother did such a thing to me. Sometimes I wonder if I hated her. I loved her for being my mother and nothing else. I tried to understand.

My grandfather always explained to me that my mother had certain problems when she was young, and she didn't have anyone to deal with her. He said that he didn't understand why my mother was the way she was, but that she was still my mother and that's why I loved her.

I was wondering how Maggie was doing. Was she happy and was she being taken care of? I remembered that she always walked around with no shoes on, and I would have to be there to remind her to put them on. She would always forget to eat her food. I wanted to get out to see her, and I wanted to tell the world just what it was like being all by myself.

I went to sleep with the thought of Maggie on my mind like I had done several times before. Loving Maggie was the only thing that held me together.

Several days later, I started to perk up and feel a lot better. They took me back to my room and started to send me to physical therapy. I started to get faster and better in school. I was even learning how to read.

The nurse then came to my room one day and she said, "The doctor wants to see you."

She put me on a stretcher and took me downstairs. I figured, "Oh, no! They're going to operate on my other arm now." But they didn't.

They took the bandages off my arm and took the stitches out. I screamed, and screamed, and screamed....

They said, "We've bent her arm, but now it doesn't move. Her bones are rigid. Wherever you put them that's where they will stay. There's nothing we can do, but further her education."

So I felt that they were going to give up operating on me. I was glad about that.

I started to enjoy myself in physical therapy. I had a Chinese therapist who was teaching me how to get around. She was teaching me how to exercise myself, and I already knew how to crawl and roll around. I had learned that by myself.

One day she stood me up on my knees. She gave me some crutches, but they weren't the right height for me. She put them under my arms and taped them there because I had no grasp. She would stand in front of me and I would lift the whole left side of my body up and lean on the crutches forward. Then I would lift my right side up and swing that crutch forward. Then I would move my knees one at a time forward.

After several weeks of this, I could scoot down the hall to my room and into the ward, and I really was walking.

One day I was coming down the hall. I fell and slid under a chair, bursting my head open. They took me back downstairs and sewed up my head.

After I recovered from that, I started wearing a football helmet everytime I walked. I started getting sores on my knees from the hard floor, and I would even wear knee pads. I felt like a real football player with a helmet and knee pads.

By this time, I was nine years old and had gone to the fourth grade. At the end of the year, I didn't have Mrs. D.O. anymore. I had Mr. Clarke. Mr. Clarke told me that I had learned so much during the year that he wanted me to skip the fifth grade and go to the sixth grade.

Doctor Sawyer came in and congratulated me for being skipped to the sixth grade. He told me that he knew I could do it, and that I had the smarts.

On my tenth birthday, my mother came to see me. Four years had passed without seeing my mother. I wasn't sure about how I felt about seeing her. I told them I didn't want to see her.

The nurse said, "Are you sure you want to tell your mother that?"

I said, "Yes, I like the place." I didn't want to go anywhere, though I sure did want to see Maggie. But they said she was too young to come and see me.

So my mother came in anyway. She was with another lady named Lucy.

She said, "Look at your hair, chile! It's almost down to your ass."

Now she was bringing me back to those words once again. I remembered that she used those words often. Next my mother pulled some money out of her pocketbook.

She said, "Do you want anything?"

It was funny because I didn't know what money was. Isn't it something to be ten years old and not know what money is?

I said, "No, I don't want nothing. I just want to be left alone."

She said, "Don't you talk to your mother like that. Come here and let me do something to your hair."

My mother combed my hair, and put some grease in it, which I had forgotten all about. She was right, my hair was down to my ass.

Mother said, "Next time I come I'm gonna cut it off. I want you to meet my friend, Lucy."

I looked at her and said, "Hi, Lucy."

Lucy replied, "How are you?"

I said, "Oh, fine."

She said, "Your mother has told me a lot about you."

I said, "Oh, yeah. Like what?"

"Like how bright you are. She say's you're very intelligent."

Lucy started asking questions like my mother should have been asking me.

I asked my mother how Maggie was doing.

She said, "That girl is getting too fresh. She has titties now. She's only nine years old."

Dr. Sawyer came in and greeted my mother. "I know you've heard a lot about Celestine's progress. She's going to the sixth grade."

My mother said, "She's not going anywhere. She's going home."

Dr. Sawyer said, "We'd like to keep her on, to see how far she can go in her schoolwork. Maybe she can come in on a daily basis."

My mother said that she didn't have time for all that; she was coming to get me next week.

I told my mother I didn't want to go home. I just wanted to see Maggie and then come right back to school to learn.

My mother said, "Don't argue, chile, you're going home anyway."

She turned and said to Lucy, "Let's get going. I have to get some things before we go home."

Remembering what my mother was like, I could imagine what those things were. So they turned around and left. I started to think what I could do at home. I wanted to see Maggie so much, but I didn't want to go home. I worried all night long.

The week seemed to go quickly. On the last day my class gave me a going–away party. I had learned to adjust to the place, and it had become home. The nurse who used to come to visit me on Sundays since my own mother wasn't there asked me if I would like for her to come and visit me at my home. I had to tell her no, because I knew what my mother would be like if I had a white lady come to the house.

When I was ready to cut the cake, my mother came in.

She said, "Ooh, good, cake! Can I have a piece?"

I wanted to say, "No," but I said, "Yes." I cut the cake with the knife in my mouth and gave everybody a piece, it was a very nice party.

My mother was dressed in a new black and white pantsuit. She put a brown fur coat on me that covered me from head to toe and made me feel like a polar bear.

She picked me up and said, "Ooh, chile, you're getting so heavy. I'm gonna take you home and put you on a diet." I only weighed about fifty-eight pounds at the time. I was ten–years–old.

I said goodbye to all my school friends and to Mrs. D.O. Without her help, I wouldn't have learned anything.

Doctor Sawyer was waiting to kiss me goodbye. It was a very sad occasion for me.

I said goodbye to the receptionist. Then my mother carried me to the car. There was a lot of snow on the ground. This was the second time I had seen snow in my life, and I knew it was cold and wet, but I could only guess what it felt like.

Pretty soon we got to the place that my mother considered home. It was a dirty neighborhood with trash all over the street, things that I had never seen before. There were people standing around in front of the bar. My mother picked me up and took me inside. The house was dark and dreary. It was real big. I think it was three stories.

Maggie came running down the stairs. There was no need anymore, for me to remind her to put her shoes and socks on before going outside. She was bigger than me now. She had long beautiful hair, just like mine. We looked amazingly alike. It was like love at first sight, remembering all the good times we had in the past.

Mom had put me down on the couch, and Maggie hugged me. I was both afraid and glad to see Maggie at the same time. She helped me to get my coat off and asked me if there was anything I wanted to eat.

I said, "No, I just ate some cake."

She said, "Boy, do I have some stories to tell you when we get in bed tonight!"

I heard my mother say, "Maggie, Maggie, get your ass in this kitchen. Didn't I tell you to wash these dishes?"

Maggie said, "I did wash those dishes!"

Mom said, "These dishes are so dirty I wouldn't eat off of them!" She made Maggie wash the dishes all over again.

She said to me, "Teeny, do you want to come into the kitchen?"

I said, "Yes," and she spread a blanket on the floor for me and laid me on it.

Mom said, "Maggie, wash, and you dry." It sounded like fun.

She put a towel on my feet, Maggie handed the dishes down to me on the floor, and I would dry them off. Then she would pick them up and put them into the cabinet.

Mother asked me what I wanted for dinner, greens or black-eyed peas. I couldn't remember those things, although I probably had them before. I didn't know what to say, so I picked peas because I didn't think I would want any greens. I had black-eyed peas, corn bread, and pork chops. It was such a big change from ravioli, lasagna, and eggplant. I enjoyed it; it was very spicy. But I got a bad stomachache afterward.

Mom and Maggie set the table in the dining room. I remembered that they used the very same dishes that I had dried. I felt good about that. They brought me into the dining room, and we all ate together.

After dinner Mom said, "It's going on 8:30 P.M.; time to go to bed." She told me there was a TV in the room and carried me upstairs.

There were twin beds in the room, one for Maggie, and one for me. There were pajamas and everything for me, too. I was glad to be there with Maggie because it seemed like she needed some company. Even with the twin beds, we slept together. I asked Maggie when she went back with Mom because when I had last seen her, she was with our grandmother.

She said, disgustedly, "Mom came and got me when I was in the second grade. I didn't want to come back here, but I didn't want to stay there with them." She continued, "All those kids around there acted like I didn't even belong. But you know how nice grandmama is."

I said, "Oh, yeah? I haven't seen her in a long time. I would like to see her."

Maggie said, "We'll probably go over there tomorrow. They'll probably want to see you anyway."

We laughed and giggled. Then Mom called out to us, "Shut that damn noise up, and go to sleep."

I said, "I remember those words." And Maggie laughed.

We finally giggled ourselves to sleep.

Early the next morning, my mother woke us up and asked what we wanted to eat for breakfast. Mom asked me if I wanted waffles, which I was familiar with, or grits, which I wasn't familiar with.

So I took waffles, and Maggie wanted grits.

So we had grits and waffles for breakfast. And I kind of liked the grits, but I loved the waffles.

After breakfast my mother's friend, Lucy, who I liked a lot and wondered if she lived there or not, said, "What time do you want to go over to your grandmother's house? Frances—I mean."

"What time does Frances want to go over to her mother's house?" she said. "As soon as I bathe the kids and get dressed."

Then she dressed us up, and Maggie looked very pretty. And come to think of it, so did I. So we were on our way to grandmother's house. I forgot exactly what she looked like, but I never forgot her sweet personality. She always liked to baby me, feed me, and do things for me that I could do for myself. I knew she did it because she loved me.

As soon as we got there, it was very familiar. The streets were clean and there were flowers outside in every flower pot. They seemed kind of dead because of the weather.

My mother carried me into the house. All these funny–looking children started jumping all over me. I was wondering who they were, but I was afraid to ask because my cousins figured I should know who they were. They all knew who I was.

My grandmother came running out of the kitchen crying, "My baby, my baby." Then she bent over the couch and started kissing and spitting all over me. I didn't like that very much, but I gritted my teeth.

Maggie really wanted to see my grandpop, too. He never had too much to say, but he was kind of nice, and he would always put me in the front seat of the car when he was driving. I felt very big in the front of the car. I had never forgotten his car.

Several of my cousins (I imagined that's who they were) began asking their mother for money. I wondered what money was. Their mother reached into her pocketbook and got these coins out. I was told that they were quarters, nickels, and dimes from my lessons at school, but I never knew what they were used for. Next my aunt gave everyone a dime and asked me if I wanted something from the store.

I said, "No," because I had never had much candy at school. I wasn't familiar with what you could buy at a store. She told them to get me a candy bar.

Then she asked my grandmother, "Where's Pop?"

"Oh, he's not here. He's doing an errand. He should be back soon. Do you want a drink?"

I was kind of thirsty myself.

Maggie said, "I'd like to have a drink."

My grandmother said, "Oh, you drink now!"

I said, "I'd like to have some water, please."

My grandmother said, "Where did she get those manners from? She didn't have them before she left!"

Mom said, "I don't know, she's been acting kind of funny since she got back."

All the kids were telling my mother that I talked like a white person. I was wondering what white people talked like. And the way they were talking didn't make any sense to me either.

The day went quickly. I got my first taste of greens, which I didn't like very much. They were stringy, and I had a hard time chewing them.

My mother and grandmother were fussing because again my grandmother wanted to feed "her baby."

My mother told her that I could feed myself.

My grandmother said, "I fed you and I'm going to feed her."

My mother had no more to say. My grandmother got down on her knees to feed me.

I didn't need a blanket here. There was carpet all over the floor. I liked that. I told my grandmother I would rather that she didn't feed me because I would rather do it myself.

She said, "Okay, if you want to do it yourself, then it's alright."

She bent over to give me a kiss and a big brown blotch dropped in my eye. And I said, "Oh, no!" I wondered why she spat on me.

My mother ran over with a napkin and wiped my eye. She said, "It was only some snuff."

I didn't know what that was. So I just gritted my teeth again and started to eat. Everybody was sitting at the table; Aunt Libby, my Uncle Craig, my Uncle Bobby, my mother, my grandmother, and my sister,

Maggie. My uncles were fighting over who was going to get the most bread.

My grandmother said, "You all stop acting like pigs and say your prayers."

Craig said, "Thank you for this food which we are about to eat," and everybody started eating.

My grandmother said, "You all don't learn nuthin' in that damn school, do you?"

Everybody just ignored what she was saying, and we continued to eat. I was so worried because I wanted to get back to school. I was crying when I first got here because I wanted to go back.

Then in comes this big, black man with gray hair and brown big-heeled boots. They looked very dirty. My grandmother said, "Here's your grandfather."

I smiled.

He said, "How's my little girl doing?" He picked me up and then threw me in the air. It was the highest I had ever been off of the ground. I didn't know if I was going to faint or throw up. He seemed very happy to see me. He gave me some money, which I didn't know what to do with, so I gave it to the rest of the kids.

My grandfather said, "Do you want me to take you home?"

But my mother said, "Lucy will come to pick us up in a little while."

My grandfather said, "I don't know why you don't go out and get yourself a man and leave those women alone."

Frances said, "I don't tell you how to live your life and I'm not going to let you tell me how to live mine."

He said, "You hold your tongue in my house, you hear me?"

She said, "Yes, and shut up."

Lucy came and got us and soon we were back home. She seemed to be staggering a little bit. I used to wonder why she kept her hair so short and combed back. On top of that her hair was slicked down, and she always wore men's clothing. I thought to myself, *My mother doesn't need a man. She already has one.*

When we got home, my mother said that she was going out and would be back in a little while and told Maggie to take care of me. I remembered that she had left us so often before. Maggie and I started to play games, which Maggie had plenty of in her room.

She said, "I hope Mom never comes home so that they can put us in a home. I can't stand her. She's always beating me. You just don't know what you've come home to."

I said, "Well, she's not going to beat you anymore, not as long as I'm here."

Maggie smiled.

Sure enough Mom didn't come home. The next morning Maggie got up and prepared breakfast. She could cook pretty well. I guess Mom taught her how, or probably she learned on her own since Mom was never home.

After a few days passed, we began to run out of food. Maggie called my grandfather. He came and got us and took us to his house.

We remained there for several years.

6 LEARNING TO BE A TEENAGER

My mother called us from Delaware the day after we had gone to our grandparents. My grandfather said that the police were after my mother, and that she could not get to Philadelphia.

My mother was a shoplifter. She used to take Maggie and I into the store and show Maggie how to put things in between her legs and switch out the store with a long coat on.

My grandfather said to my grandmother, "You better call the welfare people tomorrow so that they will know to send their checks here and not over there."

My grandmother worked for white folks then. She cleaned their houses and scrubbed their floors. She really made a lot of money for those days: $15 a day. Everyday she would give her money to my grandfather. She would come home and clean, too. She never seemed to give out. I wondered how she could hold up and drink so much alcohol on the weekends.

When I was about thirteen years old, my grandmother started going through her change of life. I remember she would start doing crazy things like turning on the water and watching it run. My grandfather would have to turn off the main valve in the cellar everyday. She started talking to the television, telling it that it wouldn't get her.

I would wonder why she was doing these things. The only solution I could think of was that she was drinking too much.

My grandfather said that she was going through "the change" I didn't know what that meant. My Aunt Libby, who was two years older than me, called it menopause. She said Momma was changing life and getting older and that when she got over it she would be back to normal.

One day I was laying on the living room floor. I guess I was fourteen years old then. I was wondering whether I was going to see my mother again or if I wanted to see my mother again. The phone rang and who was it but my mother. She said she was coming to get the kids.

I said to myself, "Oh, no. Not again!" This time she never came.

My grandfather told her he did not want her to come and get us because she was into too many things. She got on the phone with me and started talking.

She said, "You know I love you, don't you?" And she started crying.

I really didn't want to hear it, but I listened anyway. She just cried and told me she didn't mean to do the things she did and that she was only doing it for me.

Then she said that she had to make money her way, which I never understood. At that time I was getting a complex about my mother. I didn't want to see her. I didn't want to hear her.

One day I talked to my grandfather about it. I told him how much I disliked my mother for what she stood for. I told him I didn't understand it.

He said, "I don't ever want to hear you say that about your mother again. She can't help herself. She's full of those drugs."

I didn't know what that meant either, but I do remember seeing needles and funny–looking cigarettes.

He said my mother didn't know any better and that she would probably get over it, sooner or later, and that she would come back and be my mother. He said, "Regardless of what she does, she's still your mother."

My Aunt Libby came in and told me, "Teeny, I have something to tell you." She carried me up the stairs. It was a struggle because I had started to get really heavy. She said, "Don't tell anybody, but I'm having a baby."

And I said, "Oooh! Daddy's gonna beat you."

She answered me, "I know."

And I said, "Don't tell me. Let me see." And she showed me and I didn't see anything.

I said, "How do you know?"

She answered, "Threw up this morning."

I said, "Oh, my goodness, I threw up last week. Does that mean I'm pregnant, too?"

Libby said, "No. I'm going to the doctor tomorrow. But I haven't had my period."

I said, "You don't know what a period is?"

She answered, "What do you mean?"

Then I said, "How are you going to have a period? It's at the end of a sentence."

She answered, "Not that period, dummy—a menstrual period."

"I don't know what that is," I said.

"Well, I'll talk to you about that later," she said.

Later on in the day Maggie came into the house. She ran upstairs, crying. She grabbed Libby and went into the bathroom and slammed the door. I rolled up to the bathroom door and banged on it with my foot. "Let me in. Let me in."

They opened the door and I crawled in.

Maggie said, "She was sitting on the bus coming home from school and she felt wet, like she had peed on herself."

Libby told Maggie to sit down for she had to explain to us what all this meant.

I was hoping that I wouldn't get my period for I knew I couldn't take care of something like that by myself.

Libby replied, "Let me explain to both of you what this means. It means that you're not a little girl anymore, that you're a young lady."

I wanted to be a lady. I guessed when it would happen to me, I'd be walking.

Libby whispered to Maggie, "Now you can have a baby and be a mother."

I said, "Ooooh..."

One day my mother called home and asked for some money, and that was when she told us that she had a little girl named Tamojeanne.

Since my grandmother was so in love with children, she begged my mother to bring the baby home so that she could see it. Knowing my grandmother, I knew she wanted to keep this newborn baby.

Three weeks later, my cousin, Jimmy, came over. He told my grandmother he had been in New York to see Frances and the baby. He was with his girlfriend. I don't remember her name, but she was a beautiful lady.

Mom asked her if she wanted a cup of coffee and something to eat, like she did when everybody came into the house.

The lady said, "No, thank you."

Daddy used to get mad because Mom would feed everybody who came into the house. She was kindhearted that way.

Mom asked Jimmy when was he going back to New York, and if he would talk to Frances into bringing the baby back home.

Jimmy told Mom he would have brought the baby home if he knew that there was room enough for it. "Frances don't need that baby, she's too busy."

Mom lit up a cigarette and started to cough and choke. Jimmy told her she needed to stop smoking.

Jimmy promised Mom that he would bring the baby home.

Jimmy kept to his promise.

Jimmy brought home the baby. By this time Tamojeanne was two months old. I saw my baby sister for the first time. She was a pretty little girl. She was very dark. The little baby had one little patch of hair on the top of her head.

Jimmy brought her into the house all wrapped up in blankets. It was starting to get cold then. It was the first part of September.

Mom bent over and put her on the floor near where I was laying. I quickly snatched the cover off of her with my mouth. Maggie came in the house after going to the store for my grandfather.

She said, "Who's this?"

And I told her, "It's our sister, Tamojeanne."

Maggie said, "The baby is so pretty," and she bent over to pick her up.

I grabbed Tamojeanne by her shirt and said, "Don't pick her up. Bring her down here with me."

Maggie put down the bags of groceries and sat down on the floor. We all started to discuss what we were going to do for Tamojeanne, and how many clothes Daddy was going to buy her. We just knew that she was going to stay.

Libby came down the steps. Her stomach was getting bigger everyday.

She said, "Is that Jimmy's voice I hear?"

I said, "Yup, and here's Tamojeanne."

Libby came over, bent down, and kissed the baby on her forehead. She told us not to kiss the baby on the mouth because we'd give her the colic, and I told her that she doesn't have a collar on her shirt, and she laughed and said that wasn't what she meant.

Then she said not to kiss the baby on her mouth because it would give her germs.

My grandfather and Jimmy were in the kitchen discussing whether Tamojeanne was going to stay. Jimmy said that Frances needed money. My grandmother said that she would give Frances anything if she would let the little baby girl stay.

Knowing that my mother took drugs now, I was wondering whether Tamojeanne got sick from it because she kept blinking her eyes and her left leg kept twitching. I thought it was very unusual at the time.

Tamojeanne started hollerin' real loud, and Maggie started to pick her up. After she picked her up, Tamojeanne continued to holler, and her screams got louder and louder.

Jimmy came in and got Tamojeanne, laid her on the couch, and took out this little white plastic bag with powder inside. He took the powder and put it on the end of a spoon he had in his pouch.

He told Maggie to go into the kitchen and get some water. He put a few drops of the water on the spoon, and told Maggie to hold the match under the spoon. Then he poured it into a cap when it turned into a clear liquid.

I remember it well because of the effect it had on Tamojeanne.

Then he took this little nose dropper and put it into the cap and gathered up some liquid, and he put a drop of it into each of Tamojeanne's nostrils.

Tamojeanne's screams soon decreased.

After the loud crying stopped, she became very limp. Her arms and legs seemed to be dead. When you picked her up, her body would just lay. Her eyes started to turn in her head. She had a very strange grin on her face. She seemed to be happy.

My grandmother told Jimmy that he couldn't keep putting the baby through that. She asked him if he wanted the baby to grow up to be just like Frances.

Jimmy said that he was just following Frances' orders, that Tamojeanne has to be slowly taken off, that he was going to give it to her so she didn't get sick.

Jimmy told Mom she couldn't take her to a doctor because they would take Tamojeanne away from her.

The baby seemed to be fat and healthy and well fed. So when it came time for Tamojeanne to leave in about a week, my grandfather said he didn't want no baby in the house 'cause the only baby was his son. And his son was around ten years old at the time. And he had raised all his kids and his grandchildren, too. I could understand his motives.

We didn't hear from my mother for two weeks, so we thought we had Tamojeanne. My grandmother took her to the hospital, and they told her that she was going to have to keep giving Tamojeanne the drugs and decrease the dosage everyday. The drug was heroin.

My grandmother didn't know much about this, so Libby would give Tamojeanne the drugs everyday. She was taking the drugs four times a day at first, but now she was getting it only morning and night. In between doses she would holler very loudly as if she really knew what she wanted and she had to have the drugs. It really reminded me of when my mother couldn't get money to buy drugs. She would lock herself in her room and tear it apart. I felt very sorry for Tamojeanne because her cries were blood–curdling.

Two weeks later my mother returned.

She said, "I'm here for Tamojeanne now."

My grandfather had become very attached to Tamojeanne. Everytime when he came home from work, he would pick her up. We had taught her to sniff her nose at him. He really got a kick out of it.

My grandmother wouldn't let Tamojeanne sleep with anyone but her. She and Grandfather had really become attached to Tamojeanne in that time.

When my mother came to get Tamojeanne my grandfather didn't want her to go. He offered her all kinds of money, but she said, "No," that she had to have her daughter.

So my grandfather told her that if she took one, she'd have to take them all. I knew I didn't want to go to New York and live with her. What my grandfather said worked.

My mother didn't take Tamojeanne; she took the money instead. I thought to myself, how could someone sell their baby for a couple hundred dollars?

My mother kissed everybody and asked my grandfather to take her to the train station.

My grandfather said, "I gave you $500 and you can't find your way to the train station?"

She left.

We continued giving Tamojeanne her medicine until it got to the point that she would get it at night only.

One day I was sitting on the porch, and I decided to write a poem about sitting on the porch. I began writing, but it wasn't as easy as I thought it would be finding words to rhyme. So one day, the lady who brought me the books told me that poetry didn't have to rhyme to have a meaning. That helped me a lot. I finally finished my poem.

I said to Maggie one day, "Do you want to hear my poem?"

She said, "Sure," and she sat down on the steps as I recited it.

Here I lay again,

Watching people walking up and down the street.
Some look happy and some look sad,
Some look worried, and some look mad.
They all look at me,
I wonder what do they see?
Do they see me happy,
Or do they see me sad?
Or do they see me handicapped,
Locked up in my own shell?
I'd like to tell you some things about me,
What kind of bird, what kind of tree,
What kind of world I'd like to see.
I love God, He sees me.
He tells me how he sees me.
So people, people everywhere,
Tell me, if you really care.

Maggie told me it was such a beautiful poem that I should send it away and try to get it published in a poetry book.

I said, "No, it's not that good."

Maggie really seemed to like it. She told me to keep up the good work. She ran off. My sister ran track and won a lot of trophies and medals. She had good strong legs, things I wished that I had.

It was getting close to Christmas again. I couldn't sit on the porch anymore because of the snow. I was kind of afraid of the snow because I had never felt the snow.

I was laying in bed, and Maggie was doing her homework. She liked to read stories about the sexual lives of people and things like this, that I knew nothing about. So I picked up one of those books and started to read it. I was reading about a man who was raping a lady, and how he took her clothes off, stuck his penis into her vagina, and things like that. I started to get a funny feeling that I couldn't understand. I closed the book.

I asked Maggie how could she read such things. I laid there and thought about what I had read, and began to feel thrills that I just did not understand.

Later on in bed on the night before Christmas when I was fourteen, I started to feel wet as if I had urinated on myself. I knew that I hadn't. I had very good control over things like that. I told Maggie, "I don't know what's wrong, but I feel real wet."

She took the cover off of me, and said, "Your period's on."

I said, "Oh, no!"

I wondered why it didn't hurt, why I wasn't in pain.

Maggie cleaned me up and put a pad on me. I begged her not to tell my grandparents because I was afraid they would put me away. I was afraid that they wouldn't be able to take care of me anymore because of my period since it would require more work on their part.

Maggie took care of me the most, putting me on the bedpan, bathing me, and so forth.

So my grandparents really didn't have to know.

Maggie got Libby, and they were laughing at me because I was the last one to get my period.

LEARNING TO BE A LADY

Soon it was time for Libby to have her baby. I heard Libby in the bathroom. Maggie and I slept together. She was in school like my uncles. Libby was the only one home during the day since my grandparents worked.

Libby called Maggie to the bathroom. It was way before the time when they would leave for school. It was still dark out. It was never too early for my grandfather to leave for work. He always left before dawn.

She told my sister that her water bag had burst. *Here she goes again with things I don't understand,* I thought.

Maggie ran down the stairs and told Daddy that Libby was ready to have her baby. He dug the car out of the snow as quickly as he could. He took her to the hospital before he went to work.

My grandmother told Maggie to stay home with me that day. Everybody else went off to work or school. Maggie called the hospital on and off all day to find out what Libby had, a boy or a girl.

At about 1:30 P.M., we found out that Libby had a boy. We jumped, partied, and had a picnic in the living room.

When everybody came home, Maggie told them the news. Everybody was happy, especially Mom. She liked to spoil kids. I had been with my grandmother for so long, and I had learned to love her so much. I called her Mom because she's the only mom I ever had. She's the mom I never had.

Libby came home from the hospital with a light–skinned baby boy with black curly hair. I told Libby she had the wrong baby.

I said, "As dark as you are, Libby, this baby is too light. This baby isn't yours. You'd better take him back and tell them that he isn't yours."

She said that he was hers.

Later on that night, the baby cried. He was so little that you could hardly hear him. I was so tickled about the new little baby.

Early the next morning, I heard the doorbell ring. I was sleeping with Maggie. It was Saturday. Maggie liked the weekends because she hated to get up in the morning to go to school.

I heard a lot of girlish voices. They were Libby's friends coming to see the baby.

Her best friend, Helen Williams, asked what Libby had named him.

Maggie said his name was Troy Valtez Cain.

And all of Libby's friends ran up the steps to see the baby. Helen picked him up first.

I heard her other friend, Lenora, say, "Oh, let me hold him, let me hold him, Helen."

I heard her other friend Shawnette say, "Oh, let me hold him, let me hold him."

Helen told Libby that she sure made a pretty baby for being so Black.

I thought the same thing.

After all of the fuss, my grandmother wanted to take the baby to feed him. As she was walking down the hall to the stairway, I called her.

She brought Troy in and laid him on the bed, where Maggie, Tamojeanne, and I slept. As soon as Tamojeanne saw the baby laying on the bed, she immediately jumped out, rolled over me, and crawled on top of the baby. She was about ten months.

Mom picked up Tamojeanne and hugged her, and then I heard Tamojeanne's voice calling out.

Maggie ran in the room and picked her up and told her not to cry.

Daddy said, "Get your ass in the bed!"

Maggie slammed her door.

Daddy started to run the steps to beat her again, but then he changed his mind.

By this time, I was thinking that he was becoming the meanest man on earth.

My mother used to beat us the same way, but this time I understood a little better because Maggie was wrong for staying up so late.

Later that night, after Daddy had been asleep a long time, Libby came creeping in the same as Maggie did.

My grandfather heard her coming in and told her to lock the door, and not to go back out.

Libby said, "Okay!"

She came in the living room and stepped over me to get to the light. I lifted up my head and asked Libby where she had been.

She told me that it was none of my business. She asked me to promise not to tell if she told me a secret. And I promised not to tell anybody. She said that she was moving out with her boyfriend, Wink.

I asked her if she was going to take Troy with her, and she said, "No."

I told her that Daddy wasn't going to like that.

Libby said that there was nothing that he could do because she was nineteen years old now.

So I sat and thought about it the rest of the night after Libby went to bed. I was very worried about her moving out because I wouldn't be able to watch after her anymore, even though she was older than me.

The next day when Maggie got up for school, she came down early to show me the marks on her body that Dad had put there from the ironing cord. She said that one day she was going to run away from this place and that she was never going to come back.

It all reminded me of how bad it was before when she wanted to leave home. I told her that things would get better, that she would just have to learn to be good.

She said that she never even had sex, all she had ever done was grind on the wall with boys.

Libby was bringing Troy down the steps to give him his early morning feeding. Troy was about two months old by now, and was getting prettier everyday.

Libby laid him down on the rug next to me while she fixed his bottle. My grandfather had already gone to work and my grandmother was getting Lenny ready for school since he was the youngest.

Craig was in a special school since the regular school had a hard time dealing with him. Mom had to go to school about Craig several times because he failed to listen to the teachers. So they finally put him away.

There was a lady coming over to take care of us. Her name was Sis. She was an old lady, about seventy-two, but she could get around pretty well.

Libby had gone back to school.

Tamojeanne, Troy, and I were home with Sis everyday.

When Maggie came home from school that day, she said that she had to clean up because Daddy was mad at her.

I told her what Libby had said about leaving home.

Maggie said that was good because Libby was never home anyway.

So several days passed and Libby never came home. Daddy asked me if I knew where she was.

I didn't want to tell on her, but I had to answer my grandfather. I told him that she was moving out with Wink, and that she said that she wasn't coming back.

Daddy said that he didn't know what to do about these kids. He said, "They ain't nothin' but a lot of worriation. I work for nothin' all day long."

He held his head down and walked slowly up the steps.

Libby called later and said that she was coming for Troy. When she did come, she made sure that Daddy wasn't home. She came in the middle of the day when she knew that he would be working.

She dressed Troy and left.

I didn't know what to say to her, so I didn't say anything at all. I knew that she was getting older now and wanted to do things on her own. She looked kind of funny to me; her eyes they were kind of red and bloodshot, like my mother's eyes when she smoked those funny cigarettes.

I was wondering whether or not Libby was smoking them, too. It's funny how things never leave my mind, no matter how many years pass by.

Mom said to let them go. She said that Libby wouldn't let anything happen to the baby. Mom always believed that we should be on our own and as independent as we possibly could be. I think she kind of learned it from me, as I learned it from her because of my independence and doing things for myself.

Early the next morning, Sis came ringing the doorbell as she did every morning. She came in carrying her heavy bag and holding her hat on her head. She was an old nice lady. All she did was drink soda all day long.

Lenny and Maggie were running around trying to get ready for school. Sis went in the kitchen, put her soda in the refrigerator, and went to her usual chair and sat down and opened one up. Daddy had already gone to work, and Mom was on her way out the door. Maggie and Lenny left.

Sis cooked an egg and a piece of toast for breakfast. Tamojeanne usually stayed up late at night playing, so she slept late in the morning. She was still in the bed.

The phone rang at about three o'clock, right before Maggie and Lenny got home from school. I was watching "Dark Shadows" on TV. Sis told me that it was somebody from my grandfather's job calling to speak to my grandmother.

I rolled into the dining room to get the phone, and the news flashed on TV in the middle of "Dark Shadows." I didn't pay much attention to it. I didn't pay much attention to news. But this time it hit me. It was about a construction worker who had a ceiling fall in on him, and they were trying to get volunteers to help dig him out. By the time I got to the phone, the man asked me who I was, and I said I was his granddaughter. He said to get in touch with my grandmother, and tell her that a ceiling had fallen in on Daddy.

I dropped the phone from my ear and started to cry. I didn't really know where to get in touch with my grandmother, so I just had to wait until she came home

Maggie came in first and I said, "Guess what happened today?"

Maggie asked, "What?"

I told her that a ceiling had fallen in on Daddy, and that they were trying to dig him out.

She told me to stop playing before something like that really happened.

Sis quickly spoke up and said, "She ain't lying. They did call from your grandfather's job. She ain't lying."

Maggie sat down and looked very worried, but she didn't cry. She asked if Mom had called.

I said, "You know that Mom doesn't ever call. But I do know that she's at Miss Churny's."

When Lenny came in, Maggie told him what had happened.

He didn't believe it and told us that we were just lying. He said, "Ain't nothing happened to Daddy." He stuck his thumb in his mouth and went upstairs.

Maggie went upstairs to convince him. I never heard what she said to him, but I heard him start to cry.

Sis said that she was leaving, and I said okay, that I would talk to her tomorrow. She went into the freezer, got her last two sodas, put them in her big bag, and put on her hat. Then she wobbled on out the door.

Soon Mom was home. Maggie and I told her what had happened. She fell down in the chair, held her head down and said, "Oh, Lord! Oh, I don't know what I'm going to do if something happens to that man of mine." She wanted to know if they said what hospital he was in.

I said, "No!"

Mom quickly got on the phone and called his job. They said that they were still digging him out, and that they would take him to the hospital.

So without further hesitation, my grandmother put on her coat and ran out the door.

Tamojeanne was under the dining room table, playing with her shoes, taking them off and knotting them up.

Maggie started towards the kitchen and asked us what we wanted for dinner. Seemed like she was turning into a little mother to me. She was cooking almost every night, washing the dishes, and cleaning up the living room and dining room.

Soon after dinner, Maggie asked Lenny if he had any homework.

He said that he didn't want to do any homework. He punched at Maggie, and she ran and got a belt. Maggie came back and raised the belt.

Lenny said, "You're not my mother, so you better not hit me with that belt."

Maggie raised the belt and slashed Lenny one good time. He started crying and put his thumb in his mouth and started punching at Maggie with his other hand.

They used to fight real bad. Lenny was just about Maggie's age. She was about a year older than him. But he acted so much like a baby that you couldn't tell.

Lenny ran up the steps, but I don't think he did his homework.

He told Maggie that he was going to tell Mom what she did when she got home.

Maggie said she was going to do her homework, and she asked me if I had to go to the bathroom before she got started.

I told her, "No."

Soon Mom returned. She said that my grandfather was a lucky man. She said he would have died if he hadn't had his helmet on. Mom said that when she left the hospital they were still digging the concrete out of his skin. The doctor said that he would be all right. He was a strong man.

Mom went to the hospital every day when she came home from work. Soon the checks from Daddy's job were mailed to the house. Mom took every one of his checks and put them in the bank. She never used his money the whole two months that he was in the hospital. She used her own money. She made $20 a day, and she used that to feed us and pay the bills.

Her drinking started to get heavier on the weekends. I thought at first that it was because my grandfather was so sick, but it was more than that. I believe my grandmother just liked her drinking partners.

There was a lady named Miss Lucille who lived down the street. There was a lady and a man who lived on the avenue; their names were Mr. and Mrs. May. My grandmother had a few other friends who always loved to drink with her every weekend. She really took advantage of that when Dad was in the hospital. She would always feed us first and make sure that we were comfortable before she began to drink.

When Libby found out that Dad was in the hospital, she brought Troy home. She still remained with her boyfriend, but Troy was back home finally. He had gotten a little fat. He even looked like he had someone to take care of him.

He and Tamojeanne would play hard everyday. Tamojeanne was walking now, and she would hold Troy up, trying to get him to walk.

Soon my grandfather was out of the hospital. He walked very slowly into the house. He had a cane.

My grandmother was carrying a big bag. She sat my grandfather down on a chair. She said that my grandfather brought something for me. She said, "Surprise!" She pulled out a big shiny bedpan.

I had never had a bedpan before. I had always used a pot or something that should be thrown in the trash to go to the bathroom in. For the first time, I had the same kind of pot that they used on "General Hospital."

My grandfather was a lot of company to me. He told Sis that she didn't have to come over anymore. He said that he would take care of me, Troy, and Tamojeanne. He just hated paying out the money.

So Dad remained with us the next two months. It was kind of slow at first, his getting around trying to take care of us and fixing us breakfast. But he managed very well.

After a few days passed, I started worrying about where Libby was and why she hadn't come to see Daddy since he was home from the hospital for several months. I was wondering what she was into. I hoped that she wasn't smoking joints because that would make Mom real angry. Mom always said that it got on her nerves.

After waiting several days more, Libby finally came to see Daddy. She had on a big winter coat and dungarees. She looked a lot older to me, like she had been through a lot. We were always very close. She could always talk to me.

Daddy said, "You ain't doing nothing, but lying girl. You could be here going to school. When you going to get yourself together? You're turning out just like Frances!"

Libby took off her coat and laid it on the banister. She called me over and sat on the steps, and told me that she was having another baby.

I told her, "Daddy is going to beat you. Troy is only one year old. How are you going to take care of another baby?"

She said, "Troy will be almost two when I have this baby."

Libby said that she thought that she was going to come back home because Wink had gone to jail, and she didn't want to stay in North Philly all alone.

So I said that Dad would be glad to hear that she was coming home.

She said not to tell Dad, and that she was going to get her clothes. She kissed Troy and took him into the kitchen and cooked him an egg.

Daddy told her that she was getting fat.

Libby said that she was eating good.

She finally asked Dad how he had been doing since the accident.

He said that he didn't know that she cared, since she hadn't come to see him.

She said that she had been busy trying to get back into school.

Dad told her, "Stop that lying again."

Daddy seemed to always know when we were telling a lie or telling the truth.

Soon after Troy and Tamojeanne ate their eggs, Libby said that she had to go. She gave Troy to Dad because he would always holler when Libby left him. Libby ran to the living room and got her coat and went out the door. Troy hollered anyway, as loud as his lungs could.

Daddy kept telling Troy that she would be back as he patted him on the back.

Then Libby came back that evening with two shopping bags full of clothes and one paper bag. I don't know whose car she was in, but she thanked a man at the door for helping her get her things. She also brought in two lamps and a table.

Mom, Maggie, Lenny, and everybody were glad to see Libby back, especially Troy, who loved his mother very dearly. Tamojeanne was drawn close to Libby, too. Libby was the kind of person who kept the kids clean and kept their clothes on them. She was everything a person could want in a mother.

Daddy didn't say anything about Libby coming back home, but I knew that he was glad. He didn't tell her to go, so I knew that he wanted her to stay.

After a few weeks passed, Daddy was back to his old self again except for a couple of changes. His voice was a lot lower, and he couldn't walk as fast as he used to, but he finally threw down the cane and walked on his own.

Then it was back to me, Libby, Troy, and Tamojeanne home again.

One day Libby got up early and spent an hour in the bathroom before cooking our breakfast. I wondered what was taking her so long. I didn't hear much water running, only a little in the sink. She came downstairs smiling. She asked if we were ready for breakfast and what we wanted. We all had oatmeal that morning. For some reason, Libby was cheerful all day. She never hollered once.

I thought she had awfully strange behavior, so I asked her, "What is wrong?"

She said, "Nothing." She asked if anything seemed wrong.

I said, "No."

Her behavior was almost the same as my mother's used to be. I didn't smell any reefers, so I knew it couldn't have been that, but she had a strange way about her all day.

Pretty soon Lenny and Maggie came in from school. Maggie went up to the bathroom to change clothes. Lenny went in the kitchen to get some cookies and milk. Maggie called Libby upstairs to the bathroom. I didn't know what they talked about, but soon I heard them arguing.

I heard Maggie say things like, "You know what this stuff did to Mom. Why you?"

Libby kept telling Maggie to mind her business. I didn't understand what the conversation was about, so I left it alone for awhile.

Maggie came running down the steps, wiping tears from her eyes.

I asked her what was wrong.

She said nothing was wrong, and whisked by me, and went on into the kitchen.

Her smile was gone. She looked very angry. I started to ask her what was wrong, but I thought it would be better not to ask.

Libby ran into the kitchen and told Maggie that if she didn't mind her business what she was going to do to her.

Maggie told her not to tell her what to do.

She said that she was going to tell Dad when he came home.

Then they started to fight.

Maggie never let anyone hit her without hitting back. She had been hit so much herself.

Lenny sat at the table and ate his cookies as if he didn't care about what was going on.

I was very scared because I didn't want either one of them to get hurt.

I told Maggie and Libby not to fight. I begged, cried, and screamed. Troy and Tamojeanne were in the middle crying.

Just then somebody came in the door without knocking or ringing the doorbell. I knew it had to be Mom, plus it was time for her to come home anyway.

Mom asked Libby and Maggie what they were fighting about.

Libby gave Maggie one hard, mean look, and Maggie held her head down and said, "Nothing."

I wondered what they were fighting about. It took a long time for me to find out what the problem was.

Later on that evening, Dad came in from work. He took off his shoes and flopped down on the sofa to take a nap, like he did every night after work.

Maggie came down from doing her homework. Libby was sitting in a chair in the kitchen.

Maggie woke Daddy up and said, "Come into the kitchen, I have to tell you something."

As Daddy walked toward the kitchen, I rolled behind him.

Maggie yelled out that she had found needles in the bathroom.

Mom said, "Is that what Libby and you were fighting about earlier?"

Dad shouted, "I knew that you were going to turn out like that damn Frances."

It was the first time I had heard my grandfather curse, and I knew he was mad.

Mom had already put out the meat she wanted to have cooked.

I told Libby that I was going to help. I rolled into the kitchen where Libby was. I told her that after eating my sandwich, I was going to help her stop taking drugs.

She said, "Good," and that we were going to do it together. She told me that I was really getting big. I was sixteen years old now. She asked me what kind of things I think about. Did I ever think about having a boyfriend?

I told her I did, but I didn't care one way or the other, only because I thought that I would never get one.

Soon everyone was home, sitting at the dinner table.

Daddy told Lenny to get his thumb out of his mouth and his elbows off of the table.

Maggie was setting the table, and Libby was putting food on the plates.

Daddy asked Libby if she had gone to the hospital like he told her.

She told him she did, and that they had given her some little bottles of brown medicine.

Maggie asked her what the medicine was called; Libby said it was called methadone, and that it was going to help her stop taking drugs.

Daddy told Libby to be sure to take the medicine like the doctors told her. He asked her if she wanted her baby to come out like a drug addict.

Everyone looked at Daddy. How did he know that she was pregnant? I guess he had some experience since Mom had thirteen children.

Libby was taking her medicine every day, like she was supposed to. For awhile she was drinking four bottles a day. Then it was up to eight bottles a day. I wondered to myself if she was drinking too much. But when I asked her, she said that the doctors told her how much to drink.

One day Maggie and Mom were home with Libby and us. I heard a big "Ker–plunk" over my head upstairs.

I called Maggie. She was in the kitchen. I said that it sounded like somebody fell.

She ran upstairs and said that Libby was stretched out on the floor unconscious. She woke Libby up and walked her slowly down the steps.

Maggie asked Libby if she wanted to go to the hospital.

Mom looked at her eyes and felt her pulse.

Libby said, "No," and told us to quit fussing. She felt alright and we should leave her alone.

When Dad and Lenny came home from working on Saturday, Libby said that she was going with Dad to pick up my record player from the shop. One of Dad's friends, Mr. Edwards, had given it to me.

Libby asked Dad if she could drive, since she had just gotten her license. Dad usually let her drive with him in the car, so she put Troy's coat on him, and everyone else stayed home with me.

A couple hours later, the telephone rang. Mom answered it while she was cooking dinner in the kitchen.

I couldn't understand what was being said, but I knew Mom sat down in the chair as if something had happened.

I knew whatever had happened it had happened to Libby because of the fainting spells she was having.

When Mom hung up the phone, she grabbed her coat and said that she had to go to the hospital. Libby had fainted again. So Mom went to catch the trolley to go to the hospital.

I was praying that Libby would be all right. I was very worried about her because I knew that she wasn't supposed to be fainting like that.

We waited a long time for Mom and Dad to come home. Lenny even behaved that night. I knew something strange was happening.

When Mom and Dad finally got in, it was around one in the morning. Mom came in and laid her coat and pocketbook on the dining room table.

I asked her, "What has happened to Libby?"

Mom told me that she was in a coma. I didn't quite understand, but I knew from watching TV what a coma was.

Mom said that the doctors said that Libby didn't have a chance. She asked me, "Do you think Libby will live?"

I didn't know how to answer Mom. That was the most difficult question ever put to me in my life. I told her, "If God wants her to live, she will live."

Then I asked her about the baby. Mom told me that they said that the baby was all right. The doctor had said that the baby was a little bigger than they expected.

They got up early the next morning and went to the hospital. It was the first time I knew Dad to take off from work. He and Mom moped about the kitchen all morning before going to the hospital. They both feared that Libby's life was in a serious state.

Daddy told Maggie to stay home from school. They stayed at the hospital again that night.

Later on that night when Daddy came home, he sat down in the living room and told me that before Libby passed out, she said that she wanted me to take care of Troy. He asked me if Libby knew that she was going to die. He had hit me with another difficult question.

I told him that I didn't know.

Dad sniffed and started to cry. After holding his head down for a little while, he got up and went to bed.

Mom didn't have anything to say. I think she was just tired.

Who was to know that the next day was to be Libby's last day. We all got up early. Mom and Dad cooked breakfast. They went to the hospital to see Libby.

At about one o'clock in the afternoon, the telephone rang. Dad and Mom told us that Libby had a girl. She was a little premature, but would be okay.

Mom told us that Libby was still in a coma. They had taken the baby from her. It was the twelfth of February. Libby had been seven months pregnant.

Mom told Maggie to put the meatloaf on, that she would be home early. I hung up the phone and rolled to the steps, slid down, I and rolled into the kitchen to tell Maggie what Mom said. She was already putting the meat on.

The phone rang. She picked it up and handed it to me because she had meat all over her hands.

It was Dad, and his voice sounded very low. I said to Dad that I couldn't hear him, he had to speak up.

Dad said, "Libby is dead."

I cried. I remember I wondered whether or not I was going to believe him. I figured he must be kidding me for some reason.

Soon Mom came home. She seemed very upset. She sat in the chair and moaned and moaned at the loss of her daughter. Libby was only nineteen when she died. She cried at the thought of not ever seeing her again.

I knew that they weren't going to let me go to the funeral because they had never let me go before. I would always get dressed up like the rest of the family, but I would never go. I always understood. I never wanted to go anyway. Everybody went. A lot of people from Delaware, a lot of Libby's friends. I guess there were about four hundred people at Libby's funeral.

Mom looked beautiful that day. She held herself up well. She seemed to be very strong.

Dad said that they were telling Mom that they let Tommy see Libby at the funeral home. Tommy was Libby's oldest brother and my oldest uncle. He had been in jail for a long time for robbing and stealing. They let him visit the body.

Everybody went to the funeral, except for me and a few of my other cousins who were too young. We stayed home.

The neighbors were there preparing food for when everyone got back. The funeral and burial were the same day. Everyone got home around four o'clock. Everybody ate, drank, played music, and partied. It was like no one had died the way they carried on. But it was the way they carried on after the funeral.

There was so much food after everyone left; I thought about the hungry people it could have fed.

They just threw most of it away.

It wasn't long before everything was back to normal. It seemed to me that Maggie had now walked into Libby's shoes.

That night Maggie came home around midnight. My grandfather was waiting up for her. He was sitting in his usual chair in the living room. He was snoring and hawking his nose as he always did.

Maggie slid open the door slowly. I was laying on the living room floor with the blanket wrapped around me.

Maggie creeped in and said, "Shh."

I said, "Ooh, Daddy's gonna beat you!"

Maggie tried to tiptoe up the steps, but the steps always creaked very loudly.

Daddy hawked his nose and woke up. He said, "Maggie, where've you been?"

"I was out with Allen and the bus stopped on Germantown Avenue on the way home from the movies. There was a crash," she said.

Daddy said, "I'm going to crash your ass. Get that ironing cord."

So I knew that Maggie was gonna get a whippin'. Daddy was giving a lot of those lately. I understood why, but she didn't. He was afraid that she would get pregnant as Libby had.

Daddy took the ironing cord and told Maggie to take off her clothes. She refused and he just beat her with the ironing cord anyway.

She said, "Daddy, I'm not going to do it anymore. I'll be home early every night."

He told her, "I want you in the house at ten o'clock."

Maggie said, "Yes," and screamed her way up the steps.

I wished Maggie would have understood that Dad didn't want her to be like Libby.

Early the next morning, Tamojeanne came wobbling down the hall. I looked at her and realized that Tamojeanne was a pretty normal, healthy child by now. It almost seemed as if nothing had ever happened to her. But in my mind, I knew that it was something she would carry with her all of her life. If no one ever told her, I would, I vowed. I feel that it is very important that a person takes the time to evaluate what they are doing to their children, and I feel that simply because they think they have no future that they should not take their children's future away from their blessed young ones.

By this time, I knew that I was ready to become a lady. I wondered how the whole world was going to survive now. It was a very moving experience to watch Tamojeanne, and now Troy, grow together. Their childhood existed as mine did, with someone being better than the other.

Maggie was going on a lot of dates at this time. My grandfather was getting kind of worried that she might go out and do the same things that Libby did.

I watched Libby date, and now I watched Maggie date, and to have never had a date was a difficult adjustment to make throughout my life. It wasn't too hard for me not being able to play rope, or go to school, and do other things like other children. There were a lot of things I found I couldn't do as a lady.

After the confusion, all the heartache, and the pain of the funeral was gone, it left most of us but it never left my grandmother. She was a beautiful lady. To me it seemed like she had become more of an alcoholic after Libby died. She started drinking every day instead of just on weekends.

My grandfather was very hurt because he loved Libby and he spoiled her. He gave her everything she wanted, for he only wanted what was best for all of us.

One day the doctor called from the hospital and said that Libby's little baby was ready to come home. She was premature, and she had stayed in the hospital for about two weeks.

Daddy came in and Mom told him what the doctor said, but she was drinking too much to take care of the baby, and there was already Tamojeanne, Troy, and me. Daddy said maybe I can see if "T" will take her, and I asked Daddy who "T" was. He said that she was my Aunt "T," his sister.

So he called "T" and asked her if she could take the baby. Mom said, "We haven't even given the baby a name yet."

Daddy said, "It don't make no difference to me what you name her.

I said, "Why don't you name her Libby, after her mother?"

And that was her name, Libby.

I could feel myself growing up more and more every day. I was finally becoming a lady. I had more responsibility with Troy and Tamojeanne than ever. I never knew how much help Libby had given me until she left me. My grandmother didn't work too much longer after Libby's death. She drank more, and she couldn't maintain her job, so she finally came home with me, Troy, Libby, and Tamojeanne.

One day Maggie brought home this guy named Mitchell. Daddy thought they seemed to hit it off all right. Daddy just told him he didn't want him keeping his daughter out too late at night. And Mitchell agreed.

Mom liked Mitchell. She said he was a handsome young man. And she told Maggie to treat him nice. She asked him if he wanted anything to eat like she did for everybody else who came to the house.

Then later on Maggie and Mitchell seemed to grow closer and closer together, as Maggie and me grew further and further apart.

On her next birthday, Maggie was going to be fifteen years old, and I was becoming more worried about her.

On one particular evening she stayed out all night. When she got home the next day, Daddy was furious. He got the ironing cord and beat her, and he told her not to ever do it again.

She came and told me that she was getting too old to be whipped, and that she was going to run away with Mitchell and never come back.

My sister told me that when she got enough money, she would send somebody to get me. I cried at the thought of losing Maggie, like I had lost Libby. I didn't know what I was going to do now. Mom drank a lot all day with her friends, and I was the only one home to watch Troy and Tamojeanne.

Maggie called me every day and told me how she was.

One night Daddy said, "Get the cops. If she's around her girlfriend's house, we'll get her."

Maggie seemed to be too smart for that. She kept going and never came back. When she did, she had a job. She was no longer living with Mitchell. I don't even think that lasted two weeks. They had courted a long time at the house.

By this time, Maggie was fifteen years old. She had her welfare check changed to her name and had an apartment of her own.

She asked me if I had wanted to come and visit her. I told her that I would one day. I was working hard every day with Tamojeanne and Troy.

There was a lady who was a school teacher from the County Board who came over and tried to teach me how to read and write. I didn't know much, so she told me that she was going to see if she could get me into a school.

That's something that I had always wanted to do ever since I was a little girl. I never thought I would get the chance to go back to school.

She talked to some people and had them call my grandfather. They told him where to bring me and at what time.

My grandfather took me to the front door of this big hospital building. I didn't care what they did to me this time, I just wanted to go to school.

They took me on a stretcher into the hospital. We rode down a long corridor and up to the elevator. Within a couple of seconds, the elevator door opened.

"Fourth floor please," the man in the elevator said.

The orderly and my grandfather pulled the stretcher out of the elevator. We rolled down a little hall and up a big hall. In the middle of the hall there was a lady sitting behind a desk typing away. She was a small, innocent–looking lady. She seemed to be very nice.

I asked her, her name, and she said, "Is this Celestine Tate?"

I said, "Yes, and what is your name?"

She said, "My name is Suzy, and Doctor Finmore will be with you in a minute."

A doctor came out of an office, and he said, "Is this Celestine Tate?"

And I said, "Yes," again.

Doctor Finmore said, "Bring her into my office."

So they brought me into the office and laid me on the table.

My grandfather said, "I'll wait outside." Then he said, "I'm going to the car to smoke a cigarette."

So they closed the door and Doctor Finmore asked me, "How are you feeling?"

I said, "I'm feeling fine."

I asked him if they did operations in this hospital.

He said, "Yes."

I told him that I had enough operations when I was a little girl, and I didn't want anymore.

He asked, "Did the operations help?"

I said, "No, they didn't do anything for me. I don't want to be cut open no more. I just want to go to school."

Doctor Finmore said that everything would be fine. He asked me how I got around at home.

I told him I crawled around on the floor.

He said, "How do you do it?"

I told him how I wiggled my body and moved up and down.

He turned my head to the side and put his hand against my face. He said, "Turn your head back."

I turned my head and pushed, and it pushed his hand a little.

He said, "You have a strong neck." Then the doctor asked me, "Do you always lay like that on your stomach?"

I said, "Yes, that's how I get around."

He asked me to wait a minute while he went out in the hallway. He came back with three men. They were doctors also.

They all looked at me and examined me. He told them I didn't want anymore operations. "She told me so," he said. They all looked at me again. Dr. Finmore said, "She just wants to go to school."

Then the other doctor asked the same question Doctor Finmore asked, "How do you get around?"

Dr. Finmore said, "We'll show you, okay, Celestine?"

I said to him, "Call me Teeny; that's what all my friends call me."

He said, "Okay, Teeny, let's show them."

So he told the doctors to pick me up and help me to the floor. I wiggled out into the hallway and down the hall. When I got to the end of the hall, a door opened. A nice lady came out and said, "Would you like to come in?"

I looked in the doorway, and it was a classroom. I don't know what frightened me at that moment, but I told her, "No, I don't want to come in."

I rolled back down the hallway, and my grandfather was coming up. I remember being thankful that this place wasn't like the place I was in before, when I had to stay in bed all the time. Here I could get on the floor anytime I wanted to do so.

Doctor Finmore was a really nice man. I learned to respect, love, and admire him as a human being. I don't know if there are any other doctors who would understand a person's condition and let them maneuver themselves on the floor in the hospital. I got around the hospital fast, and I went the other way. I rolled down another hall, and there were some kids in a room. They were eating. They said, "This is the day room; would you like to come in?"

I said, "No" and rolled back to where my grandfather was.

Suzy told me to come into her office and stamp some papers because Dr. Finmore wanted to talk to my grandfather.

So I went into her office, and she gave me a piece of paper and a stamper. The stamper had "1972" on it, and I was stamping paper, picking it up with my mouth, and stamping the piece.

Dr. Finmore knocked on Suzy's door after awhile and told me to come out.

He asked me, "Do you like it here?"

I said, "Yes."

Daddy said, "They're going to keep you so that you can go to school."

I asked him, "How will I get my clothes?"

Dad said, "I will bring them to you."

I asked him, "Who will take care of Tamojeanne and Troy?"

Daddy told me, "Don't worry about them, they will be taken care of."

I was very happy but also wanted to go home at the same time.

Daddy gave me a kiss on the jaw and told me that he would see me tomorrow.

Dr. Finmore said, "You can go to your class now."

I rolled down the hall into the classroom. The teacher told me her name. I don't remember it now.

She introduced me to the children in the classroom. There were only a few, all of them younger than I was. There was a little boy wearing a bag. He had gotten shot, I gathered by accident. There was another little boy in a wheelchair and another boy sitting at a desk.

She asked me, "What grade are you in?"

I told her, "I don't know, but I don't know how to read."

She gave me an A–B–C book to find out if I could recognize the letters. Most of them I could, but I couldn't remember what some of them were.

She gave me a math problem, one plus two. That was easy. She gave me a fourth–grade math book because I learned how to count by counting money. But I could hardly read at all. After being there awhile, I got kind of spoiled. Everybody treated me very well. The nurses were nice to me, too.

It was kind of hard learning to get up early every morning just to go to school. The teacher was very good. I learned things quickly. I got bored after being at the school for so long without seeing Tamojeanne and Troy that I cried and told Daddy to come and get me.

They let me out on a weekend pass and I went home to see Tamojeanne and Troy.

Maggie asked me if I wanted to come to her apartment and spend the night.

I said, "Yes."

So Tamojeanne, Troy, and I went to her apartment. Troy was about two years old, and Tamojeanne was three.

Maggie had a very nice little apartment. It was called an efficiency. It had a kitchen, a bathroom, and one big room. She had a bed couch with rugs on the floor, and it looked very nice. A lot of her furniture looked like it came from a discount store, but she painted and covered it and made it look nice.

She was dating a lot of different men then. I didn't know all of them, but I got to know most of them. We had fun. She cooked spaghetti and meatballs for dinner. Troy and Tamojeanne fought over their food as they always did. Tamojeanne always wanted to eat hers and Troy's food, too.

Maggie made it very pleasant for us. She gave me a tray with a cup of juice and my food. She said she was going out and would be back in an hour after dinner.

She washed Troy and Tamojeanne and put them to bed. Troy never said much about his mother. I guess he didn't remember. But Tamojeanne asked about her all of the time. I was hoping Tamojeanne would forget too, because every time she mentioned Libby's name, Mom, always got upset.

When Maggie came back, she had a new guy with her. His name was William. He was a different sort of looking guy. There was something strange about him to me. He seemed to be very friendly. He came in and spoke up to me right away. Right then I knew that he was quite different.

He said to me, "My name is William Taylor. What's your name?"

I said, "Teeny."

He said, "Maggie, can I have some of that delicious water you have in your bathroom?"

Maggie said, "Sure, William."

He was a very handsome man to me.

Maggie gave William a tall glass of water. It was exceptionally good in her bathroom.

William said, "I can't stay long, I have to go."

Maggie said, "I'll see you at six o'clock in the morning to go to church, and I'll take Teeny, Tamojeanne, and Troy with us."

William got up and went to the door. He said, "Shalom, Maggie, Shalom, Tamojeanne. I bet you don't know what that means."

I said, "You're right!"

Then he said, "That means goodbye."

And I said, "Shalom."

Maggie came into the living room out of the kitchen, kissed William on the jaw, and let him out. She said, "We're going to go to church tomorrow, Teeny, but I don't have nothing that can fit you. Let me look in the closet."

She tried a couple of her dresses on me. They fit a little, but she couldn't zip them. I was a little bigger than Maggie. I had started sprouting out after my period.

Then Maggie started looking at some big scarves that she tied on her hair and wrapped one around me and tied it. It looked just like a dress.

She said, "This is what you're going to wear to church tomorrow, Teeny."

She got up early the next morning with Tamojeanne, Troy, and me. She dressed us all, and she was in the kitchen packing lunch when the doorbell rang.

I said, "How long are we going to be there?"

She pushed the button to open the door. She said, "We'll be there all day, we're going to New Jersey."

I said, "Oh boy, New Jersey! I've never been there before."

So William Taylor came up to the door. Maggie said, "Shalom," and gave him a kiss.

He said, "Shalom, Teeny."

I said, "Why are you saying goodbye? Are you leaving already?"

He said, "No, Shalom also means hello."

I responded, "Shalom."

He said, "Maggie, are you just about ready?"

"Yes," she replied.

William put his coat on. Then he got my coat and started to try and put it on me. He didn't know exactly what he was doing, but he sure was willing to try, and he made me feel so good.

I was really starting to like him a lot. I never understood why.

Maggie was becoming very religious, of which I was glad because it would keep her out of trouble on the streets.

William finally got my coat on after a little struggle. He picked me up and carried me to the elevator. He had to lay me on the elevator floor because I was too long to fit in the elevator while he was holding me.

By the time we got to the ground floor, Maggie was pushing the button on the elevator to come up.

William opened the door and I crawled out. He said, "Wait right here, and let me go open the car door."

As he ran to open the car door, Maggie, Troy, and Tamojeanne were coming down the elevator. William ran in and opened the door to the elevator for Maggie.

She said, "Get the bags, they are too heavy."

William said, "What are you carrying in these bags?"

She said, "Our lunch."

He said, "You have enough food in here to feed an army." Then he took it out to the car.

William came back and got me, took me out to his station wagon, and put me in the back. Off we went to New Jersey.

It was a quarter to eight. We had to go and pick up Toya and Linda. William went to Toya's house and then went and picked up Linda. He asked if we had forgotten anybody.

William said he wanted to go past his house to go get Beauty, and his sister, to go with us. His sister had a young boy named Robert who saw us and climbed into the back seat of the car with us. William went to get the rest of them.

Maggie was sitting in the front seat with William. Then William came out of the house with a nice looking, fair young lady. She seemed to be kind of hard, like she don't take no stuff. She got into the car and sat in the front seat. Maggie got out of the car and climbed into the back seat.

William got in the car and said, "Are we ready to go? It's a quarter to nine, and we should be there by nine."

Everybody was ready to go.

Beauty said, "Hi, Tameka! Hi, Toya! Hi, Maggie! Who we got back there?"

Troy and Tamojeanne were in the back with me.

I said, "I'm Teeny, Maggie's sister."

Beauty said, "Hi, Teeny! How are you?"

I told her, "I'm doing fine."

Beauty said something to William about why hadn't he come home until such and such a time last night. I was wondering how William could be Maggie's boyfriend, and also have a wife.

William said, "Don't be asking me where I've been. I don't worry about where you've been?"

Beauty started crying and acting very upset. She said, "I'm tired of you doing this stuff to me. I don't know why you do this to me. You hit me over the head with this." She was just hysterical.

Toya and Tameka were in the back of the car, where I was, whispering about how they do this every week.

I laid down and fell asleep, along with Tamojeanne and Troy. Then next thing I knew, they were waking me up to tell me we were there.

Beauty, Maggie, Tameka, and Toya got out. They were carrying the bags. They went into the big church.

William carried me in and laid me on the blanket. It was a different sort of church. William was the head of Saddler Street. He taught the people about the Bible every week, and the men rehearsed.

All of this was new to me. I loved the songs. One song I remember that stuck in my mind the most was called, "God Is Good to Me."

Soon it was lunchtime, and everybody sat down to eat. They had a little kitchen where the ladies prepared the food. They put all the food together, and we ate from what everybody had brought.

The church seemed to be more of a family church; everybody knew everybody, and I knew no one. People came up to me and started to introduce themselves.

William brought a little old lady over to me. He said, "This is so and so. She's ninety–three–years old, and she never misses a meeting."

I introduced myself, and she went and sat in her chair, where she always sat.

Maggie gave me food. Then a lady brought me some drinks. We ate well. Tamojeanne and Troy slept most of the morning until we were ready to eat.

After we ate, we cleaned the dishes, and folded up the tables and put them up in the corner. The preacher started talking again. I asked Maggie, "How long were we going to be here, and when are we going to go home?"

She said, "We should be another six hours."

I said, "We've been here all morning."

She said, "Shut up, girl!"

I stayed in there listening. I got real tired after awhile and fell asleep.

William woke me up, holding my coat. He asked me, "Did you enjoy yourself?"

I told him, "Yes, but I got tired."

He said, "That happens because we're here so long."

We were ready to go. Maggie had already packed up and was going to the car with Troy. People started saying Shalom to me and everybody around me. On our way home, Beauty and William argued and bickered as they had on the way to church.

Beauty was the first one William dropped off when we got back to the city. Then Tameka, Linda, Toya, and Robert.

Then William asked Maggie, "Are you ready to go home?"

Maggie asked, "Teeny, are you ready to go home? Or do you want to wait until tomorrow?"

I told her I had to be back at Mom's tomorrow so I would rather go home with her.

William said, "I am going to a party. Maggie would you like to go with me to it?"

Maggie said, "No, I don't want to go. I want to go home and read my Bible."

William dropped us off at Maggie's apartment. He said, "Maggie, do you got some joints around?"

Maggie said, "No."

So William pulled out some of his own.

I was afraid Maggie was smoking the stuff. I was afraid of it. I was afraid of anything with the name "drug" on it.

William rolled a joint and lit it and started smoking it.

Maggie came out of the room where she had changed her clothes, with the Bible.

Daddy came and got us early the next morning. He said, "It's time to go back to the hospital." To him it was a hospital, but to me it was a school. Maggie and I said our goodbyes, and Daddy picked me up and took me to the car.

Soon I was back at school.

Daddy asked me if I was happy at the school, and I said, "Yes, I have a lot of fun there."

When we got there, they were having an Arts and Crafts Show.

Dr. Finmore came into the room and told me he had something special for me. They had been measuring me to find out how round and tall I was. He took me downstairs and put me on a stretcher. He took me in the classroom. In the big classroom there was a funny–looking object.

Dr. Finmore told me that it was mine. It was a special wheelchair designed just for me. It's very hard to describe it, but it worked. I stood up on my knees in a body jacket inside the machine. A mechanical arm would come around from the back to my face at the push of a button with my hand.

The lever and controls would be in front of my mouth. I would control it with my tongue, by moving the lever up and down, and sideways to go sideways.

Dr. Finmore told me there were some reporters coming to see me tomorrow. I was very excited about that. I called Daddy with my excitement. I told him that I was going to be in the newspaper tomorrow.

Daddy said, "Do you need anything special to wear?"

"I don't know, Daddy!"

Daddy came over later that evening and brought me something that Mom had picked out for me to wear. It was a pretty dress, but I didn't like dresses, so I wore my turtleneck sweater with my gray and white pants.

I was rolling down the hallway of the school. In the day room there were a lot of people with cameras around their necks and notepads in their hands. The closer I got to the day room, the more nervous I became.

Dr. Finmore turned and looked at me, and when he said, "Here she comes," they all clapped for me as I rolled into the room. They were waiting for me to demonstrate how my new wheelchair worked.

Dr. Finmore was telling them that it cost three thousand dollars to make. It was the fastest and most expensive wheelchair ever made.

Everybody sat down in a seat. They started showing movies of me doing various things like eating, swimming, cooking, art, schoolwork, and things like that.

Dr. Finmore said I had a very strong mind, and that I could do anything that I wanted to do.

After they finished watching the movies of me, Dr. Finmore said that I had the determination to do anything I wanted to do.

I was eighteen years old now, and I had to go home. The hospital staff decided to give me a big going away party, but I told Dr. Finmore, "I don't want to go home; I want to go to another school."

MOSS REHABILITATION
HOSPITAL

73
ANNUAL
R E P O R T

"On May 10, 1972, Celestine (Tina) Tate a 16 year old girl, was admitted to the children's unit of Moss Hospital with the tongue twisting diagnosis of Arthrogryposis multiplex congenita—a birth defect of defective muscles and joint contractures. In Tina it meant that both arms and both legs were essentially useless. Although the disease itself is not fatal, complications resulting from the immobility it generally produces can seriously shorten life expectancy.

Tina was admitted to Moss to see if anything could be done to improve her mobility and to evaluate her chances to get an education and ultimately to work. Increased mobility—the ability to move from one place to another—was crucial. Except for a brief period as a young child Tina had never been in an upright position! She could move from one place to another only by rolling on the floor. Her condition had thwarted any attempts at formal education. Although 16 years of age, no thought had ever been given to the possibility of employment.

During her stay in Moss, Tina was given physical therapy to contain her contractures. She was taught to swim as a therapeutic tool and a recreational outlet. The Occupational Therapy Department concentrated on improving her techniques in daily living activities such as eating and dressing. The social worker and the psychologist worked hard to bring Tina out of her shell brought on by the isolation she experienced for almost all her life.

The attack on the problem of mobility was many sided. A special jacket had to be deigned to allow her to get into a wheeled vehicle and to be maintained in an upright position. The battery–powered wheeled vehicle itself was an ingenious mobility system designed by an engineering firm specializing in biomechanics and contributed to Tina by the March of Dimes.

Tina was discharged on January 2, 1973, to Elizabethtown State Hospital for Crippled Children to continue her formal education which had been started at Moss. Her outlook for the future was infinitely brighter than it had been prior to her admission to Moss. She was mobile with minimal assistance. She was potentially employable and, hopefully, could be trained for a sedentary job even though she would never have the use of her arms or legs.

The cost of Tina's hospitalization was over $16,000, part of which was paid through the Medical Assistance program and part by the hospital's own resources. We cannot forecast with certainty what Tina's future will be but we do know that without her treatments at Moss she would have spent the rest of her days vegetating in an institution as a public charge on the welfare rolls. We believe a life has been salvaged.

Tina's case was complex and expensive. She was a hospital patient longer than most Moss patients. Yet many patients are admitted each year for whom Moss is literally "a last chance". Every one of them deserves and receives the same concern as was shown for Tina, the same marshalling of the many professional skills, and the same commitment to an all–out effort. Complex and expensive? Yes. Worthwhile? Definitely."

The doctor said, "You have to go home for awhile, but I will find you another school to attend."

I had a big party. I had lobster and caviar. I didn't like the caviar;

it was too salty.

Finally my party was over. I went home, and Maggie started coming over to our house every day after school to give Tamojeanne, Troy, and me lunch.

8 GOING INTO MOTHERHOOD

Maggie called me one night to tell me she'd be over after school to fix lunch for us. By the time Maggie came over the next day to fix us lunch, it was going on two o'clock. We were very hungry. Mom set the table and drank a beer as she always did.

Maggie came with one of her friends from ICO School. She was trying to get her GED. When they came in, Maggie said, "Teeny, this is Joe. Joe, this is Teeny."

He said, "Hi!" and sat down.

Joe was a big, tall boy—young man, I should say. He was kind of fat and looked to be about six feet tall.

Maggie asked me what I wanted for lunch. I told her I didn't care, anything would do, because I was already hungry.

Then I looked back at Joe and asked him how old he was.

He said, "What?"

I said, "How old are you?"

He told me he was seventeen.

I told him, "Yeah, the same age as Maggie." Something flashed in my mind when I saw this person. For the first time, I thought about having children. I didn't understand it at the time, but I knew that time would tell all.

After lunch Maggie and Joe left. Soon Lenny came home from school, and Daddy came home from work. It was the same old day. I had decided, after staying home for a few months, that I would try to get back into another school because I knew that only six years of schooling was not enough. I loved to read, so I checked into a different school over the telephone. My counselor told me that I could go to a place called the England House, where they could transport me to school every day.

I immediately went to the England House and signed myself in.

I came home and told Daddy that I was going to go to the England House. He didn't want me to leave because he knew that I was the only babysitter he didn't have to pay. I went to the England House anyway.

After I was there for awhile, I saw Maggie every other day. Whenever she came to visit me, she would always be with this person named Joe. On one visit, Maggie asked him to go downstairs to the cafeteria and get us a soda.

When he left, I asked Maggie if she was really serious about this person. And she asked me if I was kidding. I said, "No."

She replied, "He's alright to have around, but I'm not serious about him."

Then she started telling me about all of her other boyfriends. When Joe came back, Maggie told him to help me get on the bed before they left. So he picked me up off the stretcher and put me on the bed.

I yelled, "He's strong, too."

Maggie responded that she would be back in two days to see me.

It was a nice place at the England House. I had a room of my own, a telephone, and a TV.

I met this girl named Cricket, who didn't have any arms or legs at all. She did things with her mouth like I did, and she had half of a leg, with a foot on the end. She was very nice. They introduced me to her the first day I came. I guess they felt we had so much in common. She was quiet and older than I was, but she was a white girl, about four or five years older than me.

We became the best of friends for a short period of time.

From what I gathered, Cricket's parents were alcoholics so she didn't want to go home on weekends.

We talked a lot about men. She liked a guy by the name of Larry. He was an orderly at some hospital. Their relationship couldn't go any further because he was married.

It was pretty boring in this place because it was an old folk's home, and there wasn't much to do. So I would go home every weekend. Daddy would come and get me on Friday's.

The nurses were starting to say that I was spoiled because I was the only one who went home on the weekends.

I was being transported every day from the hospital to the school. I went as far as the eighth grade.

One night when Maggie came to see me, I put on a nice pair of pants and a nice shirt. She liked to see me dress well.

When she came, she was with Joe again. He asked her if she wanted a soda. He did this every time she visited so we would have a chance to be alone for awhile.

When Joe left the room, I whispered to Maggie, "Why are you with him all the time if you don't like him?"

She snapped, "I never said I didn't like him! He's all right, but he just don't know too much, if you know what I mean?"

I told her that I liked him, and that I thought he was cute. Maggie laughed and said, "If you can get him, more power to you."

I really had something to think about that night. So I thought, and I thought, and in my thinking and going to school, soon another weekend creeped up on me.

When I went home that Friday night, my Uncle Lenny said that he was going to a party. Maggie had already gone to a party because she called me and asked me if I had any perfume. But she never came and got it, so I guess she thought she could do just as well without it.

The phone rang, and Tamojeanne answered it. She was about five years old now, and she was getting big. Tamojeanne screamed, "Joe is on the phone, Teeny, and he wants Maggie."

I told her to give me the phone. She put it on my ear, and I moved it around toward my mouth.

I said, "Hello, Joe."

He screeched, "Hello!" then asked, "Where's, Maggie?"

I told him that she told me she was going to a party.

He asked, "What are you doing tonight?"

I replied, "I'm not doing anything." My heart was pounding; I always wanted to get a chance to talk to him intimately.

Then he asked me if he could come over.

I said, "Sure." I asked him to give me an hour because I just had a bath, and I hadn't a chance to put all my night clothes on. When I hung up the phone, I told Tamojeanne to go get my nightgown so that I could put it on, and she could help me, too. Then I told her to get me the perfume. She spilled half the bottle on me.

Soon after that, the doorbell rang. I knew it was Joe. I was sort of scared, but excited, too. Tamojeanne went down and answered the door.

I told Joe to come on up. As soon as he was in the room, and he took his coat off and sat down next to me. He started to talk about Maggie. I was hoping the conversation wouldn't last too much longer.

So I asked him how had he been doing.

He said he had been doing okay.

I told Tamojeanne it was getting late, and it was time for her to go to bed.

She gave me a kiss and went into her room. Troy was already asleep.

Joe asked me, "Do you want to listen to some music?"

I told him that was a good idea.

He turned off the TV and turned on the record player.

I told him to turn off the light because the record players light shined off enough light anyway.

He then sat down on the bed next to me. He started to tell me more things about Maggie.

I told him I didn't want to hear it. I asked him if he came to see me or if he came to talk about Maggie.

He said he was sorry if he had offended me and asked me what I wanted to talk about. So we talked about ourselves. As we talked, things started to happen. Things I'd never experienced in my life.

My heart started beating so fast I couldn't control myself. No one had ever explained to me what comes next.

He put his hands gently on my face and kissed me softly on my lips. I had never been kissed like that before. That was my second beam of light, and I knew that God's plan for me was starting to take place.

At the age of seventeen, I was still a virgin. I had saved myself for one man's love. I'm sure that is what I was feeling at that moment.

Joe pulled up my nightgown and slowly started removing my underwear.

I was getting so warm. I couldn't understand what was happening, all I knew is that the Lord said that he would watch over me, and I left what was happening to Him.

Soon we were both without clothing. Here I was having my first experience with sexual intercourse. Being my first time, I knew it would be difficult. I was under the impression that when you made love with someone that they would just lay on top of you and move around. I didn't know that Joe was going to stick his penis into my vagina.

First there was pain, then there was pleasure. I felt like this was the most normal thing that I could do, knowing that everyone who was old enough was doing it, too.

Soon after we were done, Joe said that he had to go home. He got dressed and left. I didn't know I could be with Joe and feel so good.

The next day, the only person I thought to call was my sister since we were so close. I wanted to share my happiness with her. Finally I asked Maggie if she had ever waited for someone for a long time and finally got him?

She told me she knew exactly what I was talking about because Joe was there. He had already told her what had happened. She asked me how I could do such a thing to her. How could I betray her?

I asked her if she remembered what she said to me in the hospital?

She said, "Yes, but I didn't mean it."

She had started to have feelings for Joe, she said.

I hung up the phone. I just cried and cried.

Joe called me back after awhile. He told me he was sorry for what he had done to me.

I asked him what he meant.

He said he didn't mean to have sex with me, that he was just missing Maggie.

That made me feel even worse. But I still wanted him. I asked him if he could come and help me get back to the hospital because there was no one around to carry me.

He said, "Yes," and he was at my house in ten minutes.

Dad asked Joe if he wanted anything to eat for dinner before we left. He said, "No."

Dad ate his food. I wasn't hungry. All I did was look at Joe.

Joe told me that he couldn't do what we did last night anymore, because he hadn't known how much Maggie felt for him.

The phone rang. It was Maggie. Joe answered the phone. I don't know what the conversation consisted of on Maggie's end, but Joe told her to never mind, that he wanted me. I actually didn't understand what went on. After the telephone conversation, I wanted to ask Joe questions, but Daddy said it was time to go.

When we got to the nursing home, Daddy told Joe to go inside and get my stretcher. He went to the door, and brought my stretcher out. He picked me up and put me on it. Daddy told him to hurry back down because he was ready to go.

Joe told Dad that he was going to stay for awhile.

When we got upstairs, I asked Joe what he and Maggie were talking about.

He said she was sorry that he didn't want to deal with her. He asked me if I wanted him. I closed my eyes and held my head down, and said, "Yes." I told Joe I wanted to show him around the nursing home. So I took him upstairs to the fourth floor.

On the fourth floor, there was a meditation room, and there were no patients up there. It was just used for prayer. Joe took me into the meditation room and took me off the stretcher. He laid me the floor. We started to talk, then touched and kissed again.

After the love making was over, Joe told me that he wasn't ready for any children because he wanted to go to college, and the next time we made love, he would use protection.

It was getting late, and I told Joe that he would have to take me back to my room before they started looking for me.

How passionate it had become, and it wasn't as painful as the first time. Joe and I kissed. Then he left. I saw him every day after that.

The nurse came and undressed me for bed. She asked me if he was my boyfriend. I said I hoped so.

As she put me under the covers, the phone rang. It was Maggie. She told me she had talked to Joe, and he told her that he wanted me.

It made me happy to hear her say that. But her voice didn't sound too happy about it.

She said that for what Joe and I did to her, we weren't going to have any good luck.

I reminded Maggie of what she told me a few weeks ago, that it was all right to see Joe. And I told her that she underestimated me as a woman.

So I told my sister if she didn't want me ever to see Joe again, to just say so and I wouldn't.

Maggie quickly said, "Let's quit talking about Joe. We will always be sisters, no matter what. And more power to you."

I hung up the phone with only one thing on my mind. When was I next going to see Joe?

The week went by quickly. My grandfather came to pick me up after he got off from work.

Joe spent the night just like he did every week. It was a Friday night. And this is when he introduced me to the birth control method of contraceptives.

Every experience I had with him was a new one.

In trying to use the birth control that Joe had brought, I found it to be very uncomfortable that night and the rest of the weekend. Finally we didn't use anything.

Sunday came quickly, and it was time to go back to the nursing home. Joe dressed me the next morning for the first time.

As soon as we got back to the nursing home, Cricket was at the door waiting for me to get back.

Inside, while we were eating dinner, I wished I had eaten at home. They had some nasty food.

Joe sat and looked at me eat. He gave me a look that made me feel as though he could see through me.

I asked him what he was thinking about.

He said, "I had no idea that we would become so close so fast." Joe continued, "I have to figure out something so we don't make any mistakes."

Joe called the next day and asked me what we were going to do about having babies.

I told him I guessed that I would take the birth control pill.

He said he didn't want to force me to do anything, but he wasn't ready to have any children.

So I talked to the doctor at the nursing home and asked him for the birth control pill. He looked at me as if I was crazy. I guess it was because I was handicapped.

He gave me the order for the pills. I started taking them, one a day early in the morning when I took my other medication, like vitamins and things like that.

The next day when I saw Joe, he asked me, "Are you taking the pill?" I said, "Yes."

As time went on, I started to get sick and not feel very well. I went back to the doctor and told him.

He said for me not to take the pills for a week and then to come back to him.

During the time I wasn't supposed to go back to the doctor, Joe kept asking me if I was taking the pill, and I said, "Yes."

When I went back to the doctor, he told me that it was too late, that I was going into Motherhood.

FIGHTING THE SYSTEM

I told the doctor he must be making some kind of mistake.

"No," he said, "the test was positive."

They took me back to the nursing home. I knew I was in trouble now. Joe had just told me he wasn't ready for children. When he came to see me, I told him I was pregnant.

He was very upset. He told me that he wouldn't be around if I decided to keep it, and that he would rather I had an abortion. I couldn't understand why he felt so strongly about it if he loved me so much.

The nursing home soon found out I was pregnant. They told me I had to leave because they didn't have facilities to take care of a pregnant person.

The nurses helped me pack my things. Dad didn't know that this was going to be the last weekend he had to pick me up. I was afraid to tell him I was coming home for good. I really felt bad about not continuing school because it was only my third month and I was really getting back into the swing of things. It was really difficult being a handicapped adult. They make all kinds of arrangements for handicapped children, but when you get to be an adult, they don't seem to think school is as important.

Dad came for me, and I went home.

I told Joe that I was not going to kill my baby for him or anybody else.

Later on that night, Maggie called me and said she was picking me up for the weekend because ever since I started seeing Joe, we hadn't seen each other.

I said, "Okay!"

Soon I was eating spaghetti while laying on Maggie's living room floor. She told me that I was getting fat.

I told her that there was a reason for that. "I'm pregnant."

She said, "Good, because I am, too, and I didn't know how to tell you."

I asked her who was the father of her child. She said his name was Wally and that the pregnancy was a mistake.

I told her that I didn't think my baby was a mistake, even though Joe acted like it was.

She asked me if I wanted to live with her.

I said, "Yes."

I had my social security checks sent to her address instead of my grandfather's house. My sister was obsessed with money.

Soon Wally came over and they started fighting. I was so scared, I didn't know if he would hurt me, too, and all I could think about was my unborn baby.

He slugged my sister in the face, and she passed out on the floor. At that moment, I thought about her unborn child.

He stormed out of the door. He slammed the door so hard he broke the window.

Once again I found myself crawling across the floor to help my sister, Maggie.

She woke up crying, laying on my back like she did when she was a little girl.

I told her not to cry, that God had a plan for both of us.

She wiped her tears and got us ready for bed.

As we laid there talking, I asked her how she could get involved with such a violent person.

She said when they met she wasn't working, and he gave her some money to get her apartment. She didn't know that he was so violent until after she got pregnant.

I told her that she needed to do everything she could to get rid of him. So we said our prayers and went to sleep.

It seemed like I just closed my eyes and when I opened them again it was daytime.

Maggie asked me what I wanted for breakfast.

I told her that I wanted tea and crackers, that anything else would make me sick.

Maggie asked me what was going on between Joe and me.

I told her that Joe didn't want to see me anymore.

Maggie asked me, "What was wrong?"

I told her that he was totally against me having the baby.

Maggie said she knew why, but she'd rather not say.

I was really curious about what she had to say, but I didn't pursue it.

Maggie told me that she was thinking about having an abortion before she was too far along so that she could take care of my baby and me.

I told her, "Don't use me for an excuse."

Maggie said she wasn't doing that at all. She just didn't know how she could take care of me, my baby, and her baby.

I told her not to worry about me and my baby, I'd go home to my grandfather. And that's what I did.

Maggie called me the day I got home and told me that she couldn't have a baby by a man like Wally, and asked if I would please give her the money to go see a doctor.

It was a hard decision for me because I knew that would mean taking a life.

I wanted to be no part of it, but hearing the desperation in my sister's voice persuaded me to give her the money.

Maggie called me when she got to the hospital, and I kept talking to her until the abortion was over.

I felt there should have been a funeral. I feel if you are going to have an abortion, you should have a funeral because that seed also has a soul.

Maggie recuperated very quickly.

I was hoping that having a baby would be that quick, too, for it was taking too long.

Going to the clinic was very upsetting for me at first because they couldn't believe I was there for the OB instead of the GYN clinic. They automatically assumed that I wasn't there to have a baby.

Soon everyone there got to know me and they waited for the magic moment.

It was so lonely carrying a baby without Joe with me. Suddenly I needed him more than I ever did before.

I woke up the next morning and my shirt was all wet. I called my grandma to look at It.

Grandma said, "It's just milk coming out of your breasts, chile."

I was wondering why it was coming out of my breasts, but before I could ask her, she was telling me that my body was going to go through some changes I had never experienced before. She went on to say that being a mother was like being God. You are totally responsible for your chile's well–being, and it is up to you to do all that must be done. "Never wait for a man. You see what Joe did to you."

I heard the phone ringing. I knew it wasn't for me. No one called me much anymore.

Lenny said, "Teeny, the phone is for you."

It was my father. I said, "Daddy, I haven't heard from you in so long. I wondered if you still loved me?"

Daddy said that he would always love me while he was alive and after he was dead. Yes, he would always love me. He then told me he had met this girl who was ten years younger than him. Her name was Florine, and she had a baby boy which he had named Jaycee Jr., after him. Daddy told me that my name was Jaycee, too.

I said, "How? My name is Celestine J. Tate."

He said, "The "C" in your first name, and the "J" in your second name together makes J.C."

I told Daddy that I had some news for him, too, that I was having a baby. I didn't see any sense in telling him that Maggie had an abortion.

Daddy replied, "How is Maggie? Where does she live now? I want to see her."

I said, "Dad, you must not have heard me; I'm having a baby."

He said, "I heard you. It must have been God's plan for you."

I thought he was going to be very upset with me, like when that cop took advantage of me.

Daddy was very understanding until I told him that Joe stopped seeing me because I was pregnant.

Daddy said, "Where does that punk live?"

I told him where he lived and where Maggie lived, too. I was getting sick and I had to hang up the phone.

Daddy told me to take it easy. He said he was going to see Joe to see what his problem was.

I said, "Dad, don't hurt him."

Daddy said, "Don't you worry, girl. Bye."

My stomach was getting bigger every day, and one day I felt my baby move. I felt so sad that Joe wasn't there to feel it, too.

It was such a magic moment. I had no doubt in my mind that my baby would be perfectly normal because I am perfectly normal.

Later on that night, Joe called me on the phone. He said a madman came to see him. He said, "I have a feeling you know who he is."

I thought, then I said, "It must have been my father. He didn't hurt you, did he?"

Joe said, "No!" Then he asked me if he could come and see me.

My heart started beating fast again. I said I guess so, and I hung up the phone. I asked myself, "Why didn't I say goodbye?"

I called my grandmother with such excitement. I told her Joe was coming to see me. I asked her to go to my closet and get the prettiest nightgown I had.

There was nothing slow about my grandmother. She washed me and changed my clothes. Grandmother told me that I should be quiet and listen to Joe when he came.

Soon Joe arrived, and I heard my grandfather say, "Long time no see."

Joe said, "I'm sorry; I've gotten two jobs, one to take care of Teeny's baby; the other to take care of myself."

Once again my heart was pounding faster, faster, and faster. He came up the steps to my room. It felt like the first time he came to my room.

I wanted to ask him why he had come here. But then I remembered my grandmother telling me to listen so I said nothing.

Joe said, "I guess you're wondering why I'm here?"

"Yes," I said.

He said, "May I sit down?"

By this time my stomach was getting too big to lie on so I had to lie flat on my back all of the time.

Joe said that my father had come to see him and that he told me if he was a real man he would see me through this. If he wasn't a man, my father was going to beat the hell out of him. So he thought he'd be a man.

Joe asked me, "How are you coming along?"

I told him I was sick a lot and threw up all of my food.

He asked me, "Can I touch your stomach?"

I said, "Yes."

He put his warm black hand on my stomach, and I never felt my baby jump as much as it did at that moment. The more he rubbed my stomach, the more the baby jumped. Then he did something unusual. He bent over and started talking to the baby in my stomach.

I started to cry because I felt that this was the way things were supposed to be.

Joe started coming to see me every day. This made having a baby more exciting to me than before.

I wondered why I hadn't heard from Maggie for awhile, so I asked a friend to go over to her house and tell her to call me.

Maggie came to see me the next day, and told me she was going to give me a baby shower.

I was so excited. I wondered how many gifts I would get.

Maggie and I spent two days filling out the invitations. My family pitched in and catered the shower. It was very nice. I wondered why no one out of Joe's family came. I invited his mother.

I started to get angry thinking his family thought I wasn't good enough to have Joe's baby. I got so angry I went into labor at my baby's shower.

My sister ran to the phone to call the ambulance. It arrived quickly. Thank heavens! I was feeling so much pain and pressure. It felt like I had to make a bowel movement, but I couldn't.

The ambulance driver told me to take deep breaths.

I was getting hot all over again, but it was not the same hot as with Joe. It was cold and hot at the same time. My whole body felt like needles and pins were sticking in me. I remembered, yelling, "Hurry up, hurry up!" I was concentrating on the pain and nothing else. I felt I wouldn't be a young girl after this. I remembered a movie I had seen on TV in which a monster's baby jumped out of the mother's stomach. I was hoping that wouldn't happen to me.

Soon we arrived at the hospital. The doctors were discussing whether or not to give me a Caesarean section because of the position of my legs. While they were talking and I was pushing, my baby came out by herself. She was completely normal.

I wanted to see Joe, but he was nowhere around. My sister Maggie and my girlfriend, Mindy, were there. Maggie asked me if I had a name.

I said, "No, because I wanted a boy."

The next day when I woke up, Joe was staring me in the face. He said, "You had a girl, huh? Well, I'm going to name her."

I asked him what he was going to name her, and he said Niya.

Joe went out to the nursery window to see her, and came back and told me that she was beautiful. The nurse brought her to me after he left. She was beautiful.

Five days passed quickly, and finally we went home. The ambulance people put me into the bed and laid my baby next to me.

Everybody was waiting out in the hallway to see my baby. I was feeling so good. I felt like I had finally found a friend who wouldn't leave me. My baby was so beautiful! She had dark curly hair and was high yellow, as were all the babies in our family.

When the ambulance people and the nurse finally left my grandparent's house, my grandmother became so sad. She said that my grandpop told her she was drinking too much to help me with the baby and that Maggie would have to take her.

I told my grandmother that wasn't fair. Niya was my baby!

Grandmother said, "I'm sorry, Teeny, there is nothing you can do about it."

Maggie came into my room and said, "I'll take good care of her, Sis."

I started crying. I felt like someone had cut me with a knife and I was bleeding to death. I grabbed my baby's clothes with my teeth.

My sister pulled the baby from me saying, "Let her go before you hurt her."

I had to let her go anyhow for I had to scream from the pain of having Niya taken away from me. I thought to myself I finally had someone to walk places where I had never gone, and to love me enough to come back and tell me what they saw. And here my sister was taking my baby away from me.

Maggie took Niya out into the hall. Everybody was talking about how pretty my baby was.

I buried my head under the pillow and screamed. This pain was more unbearable than giving birth. I cried myself to sleep that night. I awoke at the crack of dawn, wanting my baby. I heard my grandmother stirring in the kitchen. I guess she was getting breakfast, and I thought to myself, *Maybe if I don't eat they'll bring my baby back to me.*

My grandmother brought my breakfast to me. It sat in my room until she took it away.

She said, "What is wrong with you, chile?"

I said, "I'm never going to eat again until Maggie brings my baby back to me!"

My grandmother replied, "That's foolish because if you don't eat how are you going to take care of your baby when she does come back?

I told my grandmother, "I am not going to take care of myself until my baby came back."

Grandmother said, "You're just being stubborn," then she walked out of my room.

When the fourth day passed, and I hadn't eaten, my grandmother started to get worried. She told my grandpop I wasn't eating.

Grandfather said, "If she's hungry long enough, she'll eat."

If you have ever been starving you know how great the pain is, but it did not outweigh the pain I felt when they took my baby from me. So the less I ate, the better I felt.

After one week without me eating any food, my grandmother called the doctor. At this point, she was finally afraid that I just might die if I didn't get Niya back into my arms.

The doctor came over to the house to see me. Dr. Leonard was our family doctor. He had known me ever since I was a little girl.

The doctor wanted to know what was wrong, why I wasn't eating.

I told Dr. Leonard that my family had taken my baby away from me and I wasn't eating until they gave my daughter back to me.

The doctor told my grandmother, "I would like to speak to you in the hall."

They didn't know I could hear everything they said.

The doctor told my grandmother, "If you don't give her baby back to her, this will become very unhealthy for her."

So my grandmother said that she would try to get my baby back to me.

That made me feel happy.

Soon my grandpop came home from work, and my grandma told him what the doctor told her.

Grandfather said, "That girl is just being stubborn."

My grandmother said, "The hell with that! It is going on two weeks, and this chile hasn't eaten a bite."

All this time I wondered where Joe was.

My grandma called a cab early the next morning. She said, "I'm going on an errand, and you'll be here by yourself for a little while." Then she hopped in the cab and left.

Soon she returned, saying, "I have a surprise for you." She ran up the steps faster than I ever saw an old lady run before. Grandma came into my room with my baby in her arms.

Suddenly I was so hungry. My grandma said she had stopped at the hoagie shop and bought me a hoagie.

I ate the whole thing, I was so happy that my baby was home with me.

When my grandfather came home, he asked, "Who brought this baby here?"

My grandmother said, "I do believe a mother should have her own chile."

He just accepted it.

It was so sad knowing that my sister had tried to keep my baby after aborting hers.

My baby laid next to me that night for the very first time. My mind was kind of mixed up. It was like Niya was a newborn baby to me, but she was a month old. I was wondering how Maggie must be feeling; first I took Joe, then I took her baby, or so she thought.

I felt like I would never forgive my sister, but I knew the Lord was with me, and I would find forgiveness somewhere and share some with her.

The next morning my sister was knocking on my door. She was yelling, "Let me in, that's my baby!"

My grandmother opened the door. I didn't want her to do that because I felt like I wanted to fight my sister, but I couldn't. I started to panic. I even thought that my sister was going to try and take Niya away from me again. Then I remembered God said he would always be there with me, so I wasn't scared anymore.

Maggie came running up the steps, burst into my room, grabbed Niya, and sat on the side of my bed. She took out her breast and put my baby's mouth to it. I knew then my sister had a problem.

Maggie asked me why I didn't ask her if I could keep her baby overnight.

My grandma came into the room. I told grandma that Maggie had said my baby was her baby.

Momma said, "The abortion must be getting to that poor chile." She went over to Maggie and knelt down. Grandma told Maggie that her baby died, and that this baby was my baby.

Maggie told Momma she knew that, but she wasn't sure.

Momma told Maggie, "You need to go to therapy."

Maggie laid my baby next to me, kneeled down on my bed, and started crying. She said she was sorry she took my baby, but she honestly thought it was hers. Maggie continued to say she loved me and that I would always be her sister.

I guess Maggie took Momma's advice because I didn't see or hear from her again until I went to court.

It was now lonely, but I dealt with it. I thought it was going to be difficult to take care of my baby, but my Momma helped me out. She had stopped Niya from drinking so much milk.

By the time Niya was four months old, a lady from the Department of Public Welfare came to see me. Her name was Judy. She appeared to be a very friendly person. I kind of liked her. Judy came to see Niya and me everyday. She would sit in the rocking chair in my room and rock Niya back and forth like Niya was her own baby.

I thought this was strange, but I understood. Judy had no children, and I said to myself there was no sense in stopping Niya from enjoying being rocked and held because I couldn't do it.

Judy would leave my house around 2:30 P.M. every day. When she left Niya started to cry and scream. I couldn't control it. She had become accustomed to being rocked.

My grandmother said, "That woman done spoiled your chile."

The next day when Judy came over, I told her she couldn't come over every day anymore.

Judy asked me, "What is the problem?"

I told her when she rocks my baby and leaves, my baby is still looking for someone to rock her, and I can't rock her.

Judy told me I had no right to keep the baby from her.

I knew right then she must be crazy. I called my grandmother to get her out of our house.

My grandmother said, "It is time for you to go, Judy."

My grandfather and I were having arguments then. I told him I couldn't pay him as much rent anymore because I had to take care of Niya.

Judy said since we couldn't come to some kind of agreement that she was going to send me to court. I told her I didn't want to go to court, and that I didn't believe in all that stuff.

One month later, I got a letter in the mail telling me to come to court for child neglect. I put the letter in the drawer, hoping that the whole situation would go away. Judy called me up the next day and asked me if I got the letter.

I told her, "Yes." I didn't tell Daddy because I just wished that the whole problem would go away.

Judy called Daddy and told him what she had done, and he asked me for the letter. He told me, "Don't worry, they're not going to take that baby away from you!"

I was so worried about them taking Niya away from me that I cried the whole night. I got up early the next morning to feed Niya her breakfast. She had egg yokes and bacon baby food.

I started talking to Niya, telling her how much I loved her, and that I wouldn't let anybody take her from me because she was all that I had.

I put her washrag in my mouth and wiped her face. Something had told me that they were coming to get her soon, and what could I do about it?

I covered Niya's nose and mouth so that she couldn't breath. I was thinking that I should take her away before they took her away from me. The longer I held my mouth over her, the worse the ringing in my ear became. I opened my eyes and saw my four–month–old daughter's eyes pop out. Her face was turning red as a beet. The ringing got so loud I couldn't stand it and I let go. God didn't want me to do it that way. I remember Him telling me to have faith in Him and in all that He does.

I picked Niya up with my teeth and turned her on her stomach to try to help her breathe. As soon as Niya calmed down, and stopped coughing, the doorbell rang. I heard the social worker's voice. She said she was coming to take Niya until we went to court.

They had about seven police cars to help her take one baby. My grandmother was screaming, hollering, and cussing, saying things like, "You can't take that baby, it ain't right!"

My girlfriend, Mindy, ran down the street to tell Daddy what they were doing.

They came upstairs into my room where Niya and I were laying in the bed. It was early and I still had my nightgown on. I was holding onto Niya's shirt with my teeth. I was crying and begging them not to take her away from me. I don't know if the welfare lady was ashamed or not because she sent up a policewoman. I did not even see the face of the lady from the welfare bureau.

The policewoman picked up Niya and told me, "Let go of her before I hurt you." She wrapped Niya up in her coat and took her away.

They didn't even give me a chance to say that she was sick and needed her medicine.

I could hear Daddy's voice after they took Niya out of the room. He couldn't understand what they were doing.

I wanted to holler and scream, but I wanted to hear what Daddy had to say, too.

Daddy asked them what they were doing. I could hear the social worker tell Daddy, "The judge said to take the baby out of the house until the court day next Friday."

Daddy said, "All right, I have to obey the law, but I'll get her back." Daddy came upstairs to comfort me. I told him I didn't want to hear it, I just wanted to be alone.

They kept my baby for a week. I felt like someone had taken my heart out of my body and stomped it in the ground.

For the first time, I didn't only feel just like a handicapped person, but I felt helpless, too. I wished that I had taken her life like I started to do. I started asking myself, "Why me?"

Two days before we went to court, they gave my daughter back to me. I had called Niya's Godmother, Beverly. I told her I had to go to court in two days, and that I wanted her to take me.

She asked me, "Why do you have to go to court?"

I told her they said I couldn't take care of Niya.

"So that's what they call child neglect," she hollered.

She told me to call a radio talk station in Philadelphia, and tell the public what the State was trying to do to me. I stayed on the phone practically all day trying to get through, but the line was busy.

I called Beverly back to tell her that I couldn't get through. She told me to keep trying. So I hung up the phone and called the station again. The line was now clear. I started to panic, not knowing what to say.

I heard a man say, "This is Your Friendly Talk Station."

I said, "Hello, my name is...."

He said, "You are not allowed to give your name on the air." He asked me what my problem was.

I said I was handicapped and I didn't have the use of my arms or legs. I continued to say that the Department of Public Welfare wanted to take my baby away from me. I begged him to help me. He asked how he could help me. I told him I wasn't sure.

I told him my friend Beverly told me to call and talk to Irv Homer of WWDB because he was the best.

He told me that there was nothing he could do for me. He said he was glad I listened to his station.

I hung up the phone and cried.

The next thing I knew, I heard "This Is Your Friendly Talk Station." And a lady said, "Hello. You know that handicapped lady you just talked to, I think you were very rude to her."

All afternoon every telephone call was about me. And the man asked over the air for me to please call the station back. Irv Homer was truly being sincere.

I tried for another hour, and finally I got to him again.

He asked me if I needed anything for the baby, or any transportation to court. And then he asked me for my name and phone number off the air. He had begun a miracle!

As soon as I hung up the telephone, it rang again. A man said, "Hello, may I speak to Celestine Tate, please?"

I said, "Speaking."

He said, "I am Mr. Tizdale. I'm from the newspaper. I would like to come and do a story on you and your daughter."

I asked, "When?" By this time, the fear of me losing Niya was fading away.

He asked me if an hour from then would be too soon.

I told him, "No, that would be fine."

I called Beverly to tell her the man from the newspaper was coming, and I asked her what I should say.

She told me to just be myself and tell them what the Public Welfare people were trying to do to me. She said to call her back after they left.

I only had an hour to get Niya and myself dressed and to get the room in order because Tamojeanne and Troy were always coloring and drawing, leaving their crayons all over the floor.

It seemed like only five minutes before the doorbell rang. I was really nervous to be interviewed for the newspaper.

I heard someone say, "He's from Etin Newspaper." I heard my sister, Tamojeanne, tell him to go upstairs and turn left.

He said, "Are you Ms. Tate?"

I said, "Yes."

He came over and kneeled down to my bed and asked me if this was my baby, Niya.

I answered, "Yes."

He said, "Do you mind if I take a few pictures and ask you some questions?"

I said, "No."

He started asking me things like who was the baby's father and was he participating in the custody hearing.

I told him I would rather not talk about the baby's father because he didn't take part in our lives anymore.

Then he started asking me questions about if I had finished school, and what would it do to me if they took Niya away?

He was showing me the kind of things they were going to ask me in the courtroom.

I answered the best I could, and he said it would be in the next day's newspaper.

Two days later we went to court. Maggie was there; Niya's Godmother, Beverly; and my grandmother and grandfather were with me. My grandfather had hired his own lawyer. The State had appointed me a lawyer.

They carried me into the courtroom on a stretcher and laid me up on the table.

The judge came out of his chambers and sat in the chair.

The man said, "Judge Edward Rosenburg presiding; please be quiet." Everybody sat down.

He said, "Hi," to me.

I said, "Hello."

He asked me if I knew why I was in the court.

I told him they didn't think I could take care of my baby and they wanted to take her from me.

The judge said, no, the main interest is the welfare of the child, and whether or not I could handle her care.

The judge asked the court to bring the baby into me. They laid her on the table in front of me. I pulled her pants down and took off her diaper with my mouth, as I did at home every day. It was no big deal to me. They looked at me with amazement. I changed her diaper. I pulled her pants back up, picked her up by my teeth, and turned her back over on her stomach to get her pants up in the back.

They took my baby back out of the room. The judge asked the Welfare Department to present their case. The lady from the hospital where I had my baby got on the stand. She told the judge we were having problems at home, and that I had called her crying and very hysterical.

My lawyer first asked me to be cool because I was getting upset.

Then the lady from the Department of Welfare who had visited me got on the stand. She said that our house was in such a bad state that the floor had dirt on it, and that it was knee–deep in all these things.

She lied because we had carpet on the floors. The house wasn't as clean as it could have been, but it was nothing like ghetto life or anything like that.

They asked me if I had anything to say.

I told the judge that I had plenty of opportunity to have an abortion, but something in my mind and my heart told me that it wasn't right. I told him that I loved my daughter very much, and that she was my purpose for living, and if he took her away from me, I would be all by myself again. I told him that I loved her, and that I cared enough for her. Also I could change her diapers, feed her, and do all the things that a loving mother could do in my condition.

At that moment, I remembered Beverly telling me to tell the Judge that my baby never had a rash during the entire four months of her life.

The judge said he was fully aware of that, and he was going to take his time and try and make the best judgment for the baby. He said he thought that I was a very brave person and that he respected me for my courage. He then said we would come back to court on March 30, 1976, and he ordered me to be seen by a psychiatrist.

Two policemen came back in. They put me on a stretcher and carried me back to the waiting room. I waited for Daddy and Mommy to finish talking to the Judge.

Maggie came in and asked me how things had went.

I told her that I believed things had gone okay because the Judge smiled at me and winked his eye. I was very confident they wouldn't take my baby away from me.

Daddy and Mommy came in and said we were ready to go now. The policemen came, and put me back on the stretcher, and carried me out.

There were a whole lot of people outside. It really surprised me to see a local TV news crew waiting to talk to me. The policemen were carrying me downstairs to get into the car. About three hundred people rushed up and started throwing different questions at me. I was really kind of happy because of all the attention, but I was still very nervous.

The reporters asked me questions like, "What was the expression on the Judge's face when you changed your daughter's diaper in the courtroom?"

I told them I did not look for the judge's expression because I was doing something I normally did every day.

One reporter asked me, "Do you think they will decide to take your baby away from you now?"

I told him I couldn't be sure, but if he had any feelings, he would give me a chance to try and do it myself.

Then the policemen said, "Break it up, break it up," and took me to my grandfather's station wagon.

The cameras were still flashing, and the reporters were still shouting questions at me. They put me in my grandfather's car, and we drove off. My grandfather turned on his radio, and they were still talking about me on it.

My grandmother sat in the front seat with my baby in her arms.

As we pulled up to the door, there was a black limousine parked in front of the door. Daddy got out of the car and opened the back door of the car. A man came around to the car, and told me his name was Douglas Patterton. He said, "I'm from *Jet Magazine*. I would like to do a story on you and your baby."

My uncle picked me up and carried me into the house. And the two men from *Jet Magazine* came in behind us. One man had a camera, and the other one had a note pad and a tape recorder.

I asked them, "What do I have to do?"

He said, "Just answer a few questions, and let us take some pictures. I heard you can change your baby's diaper, and I would like for you to do that for us, too."

My grandfather asked him, "How much money are you going to pay Celestine?"

The man asked Daddy how much we wanted.

Daddy asked them how much do they usually pay people who do stories like this.

I butted in and said, "One thousand dollars."

The man said, "I don't know about that. May I use your phone?"

Daddy said, "It's in the kitchen, and if you make any long distance phone calls, you're going to pay for them."

I watched the other man set up his camera equipment. After my grandmother had finished taking Niya's clothes off, she laid her next to me, where I was laying on the couch.

The man on the phone came back into the sitting room. He told my grandfather that his boss said they couldn't give me one thousand dollars, but they could give me seven hundred. He said, "Your check will be in the mail sometime next week."

So I did things like change Niya's diaper, feed her, and myself, and dialed the telephone with my tongue.

After the interview was over, the telephone rang and it was Joe. He asked me how Niya and I were doing. He said he saw us on TV, and he asked if he could come and see our daughter.

I told him I wouldn't stop him from seeing her because my own father meant so much to me.

He came over later that night and bought Niya a case of baby food and a swing. He went over to Niya, picked her up, and said she was getting big. He went on to say that the news reporters came to visit him on his job. He said he didn't want to be in the newspaper and could I please tell them not to bother him.

I told him I didn't tell the news reporters or anyone else who Niya's father was. I told him I couldn't control the fact that they wanted to know who the father was, and why the father didn't care. I knew he wanted to protect his own family because they had given me the impression that they were too good for me. At least that is what I felt when we were going together.

Two days later, a short white man, dressed in a checkered suit and wearing thick glasses came to see me. He said he had been ordered "to counsel" with me.

I told him I was expecting him, and I asked him to please sit down.

Dr. Lipperman was his name. He took out these funny looking pictures and asked me, "What do you see?"

On the first picture, I told him I saw a man with no arms, the sun was shining in the East, and he was walking in the west.

He said I was exceptional, that he knew the man in the picture had no arms, but he didn't know that the man was walking West and the sun was shining East. He thought that was very smart of me. He saw no reason why I couldn't keep my baby.

After he was done testing me, he asked me why did I want to continue to be a mother knowing how difficult it was.

I responded by saying, "It is no more difficult for me being a mother than me being me."

Then he said, "I have a good report for the judge, and it was a pleasure meeting you," and he left.

A week later the *Jet Magazine* came in the mail. I took my teeth and tore the envelope open, excited to see what they had to say about me. I turned the pages quickly with my tongue, but the book kept closing. I opened the magazine to the middle, turned it over, and smashed it down with my chin so it would stay open. I turned a couple more pages, and there I was, with my baby under my chest.

They titled my story, "Life Style." And in with the magazine was my check. My whole family called me that day to say they saw me in *Jet Magazine*.

I really felt proud. I was now being recognized for who I was instead of what I looked like. I was always proud of myself because I knew in my heart I was here for a purpose.

Time passed quickly, and I was ready to go to court again. The judge told me he was going to put my daughter under the partial custody of my grandparents.

During this time, a lot of people became aware of me. I was on national television, radio, in many newspapers, and magazines. My story was worldwide. I received seventeen thousand letters from different people.

I didn't get a chance to answer all the people who wrote to me. And I hope that my determination gave strength to those who believed there was no future for them. I feel that God gives all of us a purpose to do what has to be done. And if we would all take the time to read the Bible, we would find the purpose that he has set for us.

Search your heart, and find your dream. Dreams really do come true.

What happened to:

Frances Tate—Hasn't been seen since....
Maggie—Is still trying to find herself.
Momma (Father's Mother)—Deceased, but always on my mind.
Sandy—Left my mother and went to nursing school.
Mr. Miletti—Deceased. He was a nice man who took quick baths.
Cops—I guess police are still being police.
Daddy (Mr. J.C. Tate)—Deceased. Finally having peace.
Aunt Anita——Still being Anita with all her little crew.
Lloyd—A young man left alone. I hope he finds his way home....
Rose—All grown up with her own crew.
Rusty—He is confused, unable to choose the lifestyle of who he wants to be....
Hank—He grew like a weed and planted a seed. Now he's a daddy, and I am so happy....
Adrian—A teenage mother needing someone to hold, dealing with the burden of a lot of heavy load....
Freddy—Freddy was the oldest, but he wasn't the coldest. He was quite nice. Now he's working both day and night.
Bertha Mae—She is a young woman with a child of her own. Never can sit still, always ready to roam....
Aunt Silvia—Momma died. Now she is the Momma, sitting in the window cooling as the wind blows....
Miss Hippo—God put her to rest with all her children finally by her side. It is a shame it took her death to bring them all back together again.
Jimmy—He was the kind to take it to the limit. He was very bright and not very timid....
Daddy Cain (Mother's Father)—He's living in misery, with no plans for his history.
Mom (Mother's Mother)—She's now gone. I felt so alone, but living without her lets me know I can live when anyone goes....
Bobby—He went astray finding himself with nowhere to lay. I wish I could find him. I would ask him to stay....
Libby—She died and I cried. She left two kids behind for me to mind....
Craig—In and out of jail with no money for bail. Always trying to get a

buck, only living on luck....

Lenny—Standing on the corner drinking his wine. Spending lots of money and wasting his time ....

Dr. Sawyer—I never knew what happened to the Doc; all I know is I wish him luck....

Mrs. Desedaris—Teaching by day and preaching by night. Always thought she was a wonderful sight....

Lucy—I loved Lucy because she was true to me....

Tamojeanne (or Tammy)—Tammy had a baby when she became a lady. Always keeping a job, staying away from the rest of the mob....

Troy—He's a young boy who misses his mother, but he tries his best to keep it undercover....

Wink—Still in jail without bail. No one comes to see him, or even tries to please him....

Miss Lucille—Always trying to make a deal. She's so nice I wouldn't think not to help her twice....

Libby—Little Libby for who I feel no pity, thinks she's smart and always throws darts....

Mitchell—Mitchell went away. I don't know where. Sometimes I just see him and stare....

William—He was a man with a master plan who taught me how to understand, how to follow through with all my plans....

Joe—He went away and came back today. I know he is going to leave. I don't expect him to stay....

Cricket—She was my friend who came and went, in and out of my life....

Jaycee—The little brother I never knew; someday I knew I would....

Niya—Niya, my child, my life, and my love. I know when I die, I'll see you from above....

Beverly—Beverly was a friend of mine who I hope will stay around all the rest of my time....

Judge Edward Rosenburg—I met a judge. He became my friend, and I'll be his friend until the end....

To My Readers:

If you liked Book One, you'll love Book Two. Here's a little something from the bottom of my heart to you. As long as love lasts that's how long I'll think of you.

Love,
Celestine Tate

LETTER FROM THE AUTHOR

My life has written my book. Even as a young child, I dreamed about someday telling my life story because I am not here by accident. I am here for God's purpose.

I've been down many different roads. On some I had to turn around. Writing this book has brought me back on the right track. I hope for those who have been down many different roads like me that you will turn around after reading my book and will get back on the right track.

If you like *Some Crawl and Never Walk*, you'll love my next book. This true life story will enhance your desire for achieving all yours dreams, and giving you the will to go on with your life.

With all my love to you,

Celestine Tate Harrington

My mother has gone away.
In my heart I thought she'd stay,
It didn't matter to me that she was gay.
All I knew was that I loved her anyway.

There will be a small reward, and lots of blessings, for the person who can lead me to my mother, Frances May Tate, whether she be dead or alive.

Last seen she was in Harlem, New York, until 1986. Then she moved to Brooklyn, New York, where I lost her trail. You can contact me through: Dorrance Publishing Co., Inc.

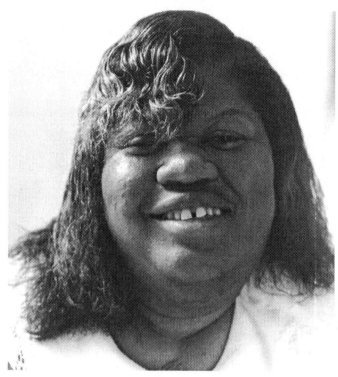

Celestine Tate-Harrington
October 15, 1955—March 25, 1998

Celestine Tate-Harrington, who was born with arthrogryposis multiplex congenita, a birth defect of defective muscles and joint contractures, won, against all odds, her case as a single mother against the welfare department to keep her daughter and went on to become a well-known and well-loved fixture on the Atlantic City Boardwalk. She died tragically on Wednesday, March 25, 1998, as a result of injuries she suffered when she was struck by two cars in Atlantic City, New Jersey. Celestine was forty-two years old.

Celestine used a bright-yellow, battery-operated hospital gurney for transportation. She had been maneuvering her gurney down the middle of Pennsylvania Avenue between Mediterranean and Baltic Avenues in Atlantic City when she was struck by the first vehicle. When she was struck by second vehicle, Celestine was thrown from the gurney. Celestine fought for her life valiantly in the hospital for six days before she succumbed to her injuries.

Since *Some Crawl and Never Walk* was first published in 1995, Celestine Tate has gone on to achieve many things.

In July 1996, Celestine's daughter, Nia, married Ernest Ball III, at Sanctuary Church of God in Christ in Philadelphia, Pennsylvania. *JET* Magazine carried the story on the front page to the delight of many of their readers who had followed Celestine's story. As a gift to her daughter and new son-in-law, at their wedding Celestine used her tongue to play the theme from *Love Story* on her portable organ. "It's my gift to them. I hope that their love can continue on for years." At the time of her death, Celestine had just celebrated her own sixth wedding anniversary with her husband Roy Harrington. She received the Martin Luther King Drum Major Award For Human Rights in 1996.

In January 1998, Celestine officially and proudly joined the working world when she was hired by McDonald's in Atlantic City where she delivered flyers and also processed telephone orders for delivery, wearing a headset and entering the orders into a computer. She wore a device on her head that enabled her to enter the information into the computer by bending her neck and pointing with her head. When she received her first paycheck, Celestine did not cash it. Instead it was framed and displayed in a case near the McDonald's entrance.

Celestine had been working on her second book, which will be completed by her daughters, Nia and Coronda.

The Celestine Tate-Harrington Memorial Fund has been established for her children: Nia Tate-Ball, Coronda Tate, and Charles Graves.

Despite her disability, Celestine accomplished so much in her life, and her moving story has inspired very many people. Even though she will be greatly missed, she continues to touch people every day. At the time of her death, both Nia and Coronda were pregnant and expecting baby girls. Nia delivered first, and as a tribute to her mother, named the baby Celestine so her name and legacy will live on.